D0948972

Interns: From Students to Physicians

This volume is published as part of a long-standing cooperative program between Harvard University Press and the Commonwealth Fund, a philanthropic foundation, to encourage the publication of significant scholarly books in medicine and health.

Interns

From Students to Physicians

Emily Mumford

cf A Commonwealth Fund Book
Harvard University Press
Cambridge, Massachusetts
1970

69140

To Harry Reiss, M.D.

Preface

Because this study has spanned some ten years, I owe thanks to many people, some of whom I met long ago but still remember warmly. Interns and residents in many hospitals took time out of busy days to be interviewed and to volunteer information. Their interest and friendly, good-humored acceptance of the observer made most of the observation and interviewing for this study rewarding and interesting.

Patricia L. Kendall taught me much through precept and suggestion when I worked with her at the Bureau of Applied Social Research. She and Mary E. Weber Goss read the first drafts of the original intern and resident study which then developed into my doctoral dissertation. George G. Reader arranged for my initial entry to study in hospitals. His knowledge of medical sociology as well as of medicine and medical education, his wide acquaintance with medical people, and his encouragement upon reading my second draft, were all essential aids in the course of this study.

Robert K. Merton, who guided the larger project, inspired and directed us as we worked, read the second draft of this report, and then the final doctoral dissertation. His generous notations and comments gave me a rich store of directions and possibilities for investigation and the courage to expand the original study.

Edgar L. Geibel and Helen Whitelaw were each thoughtful, interested, and friendly beyond any formal requirements of their positions in one of the first hospitals I studied. Charles

Arter, Jr., was another who contributed much to my understanding of the intricacies of hospital administration and the recruitment of interns. He provided the chart that compares the ten years' recruitment experience of six hospitals in one community.

Many other people contributed significantly to the development of the early study, both with intelligent criticism and encouragement. Among them, I am deeply grateful to Leonard M. Marx, Christine McGuire, Lawrence Fisher, Roger Crane, Terry Rogers, and John Hubbard. They each saw the early drafts.

The study could not have been extended without the considerate interest, time, and very real help of Ann Orlov, Robert Ebert, and Terrance Keenan. Dean Ebert, in a single meeting, added scope and comprehension to some issues in medical education in hospitals, and he helped to make possible additional field visits which were extremely useful. Quigg Newton's positive response to my request for help from the Commonwealth Fund was essential, and I hope the outcome justifies the trust.

Rose Laub Coser's incisive and detailed comments, her good questions, and sociological insights have taught me much, and her approach to the manuscript has made me proud to be a sociologist. M. Ralph Kaufman's knowledge and interest in medical education is an inspiration to me, as it is for many others who have had the privilege of working with him and seeing him teach.

Among more than one hundred physicians who have been especially helpful and very rewarding to interview, I am particularly indebted to the following: Hugh Luckey, Walter J. Zeiter, H. S. Van Ordstrand, Ralph Wieland, Charles H. Rammelkamp, E. M. Chester, S. Wolpaw, V. Vertes, Thomas Daniel, Daniel Holden, Thomas Chused, Lawrence Weed, William Marine, James Strickler, and Verne Schwaeger.

Virgie McGuffee's extraordinary talent for library research, her attention to details, ability to organize data, references, and her own work have helped beyond measure. She is a superb research assistant.

Faults and shortcomings of this book are mine alone and where they exist it is in spite of the good will and intelligence of the people I have named.

Emily Mumford

New York City
July 1969

Contents

Tables

Figures

Interns

Introduction

What happens to the person on his way to becoming a physician and as he first takes primary responsibility for his patients is of critical moment for the patient today and a large concern for us all tomorrow. Medical educators and their students assume that where one takes house-staff training is a matter of consequence. There is competition for intern and resident appointments to some hospitals, but competition for applicants at other hospitals. A professor in medical school may spend considerable effort urging an exceptional student to take his internship in one hospital but not another. The National Intern Matching Plan (NIMP) processes approved hospitals' selection of applicants and medical students' choices of hospitals to increase the chances that the particular hospital and medical student will be well met.

The American Medical Association's "Millis Report," *The Graduate Education of Physicians,* recognizes the potential impact of house-staff experiences and urges study of intern and residency programs. These have multiplied and lengthened without over-all planning and design. Too little attention has been paid to the continuity and coherence of the total years of medical education through residency.[1] Too little comprehensive planning has attended to ways to produce the variety of physicians that the nation urgently needs.

The internship stage of training offers a nearly perfect example of potentially effective adult socialization. The beginning physician is introduced and moved into patterns of behavior with his colleagues and with patients in an emotionally charged atmosphere. His encounters and experiences there can reinforce and protect some of the commitments he began to form in medical school. Or he can face a series of frustrations, reality shocks, and contradictions, as well as escape routes that provide alternatives and possibly rationalizations for altering the commitments. The years of house-staff training often provide a physician's first personal encounter, his initiation rites, in medicine. For some, these years are also the last chance the medical profession has to exert direct, sometimes round-the-clock, and near-exclusive influence or control.

Many interns I have met come to their house-staff training with obvious eagerness and concern. They are attentive to their first patients. They are open, hopeful, and willing doctors—and not a few of them are vulnerable. Some show almost touching candor and lack of pretense. Two interns, on their first meeting, described their efforts to gain entry into one internship program. One explained, "I didn't think they'd have me. I feel lucky to be here." All the American-trained house-staff members have shown enough interest in becoming physicians to study and take exams, first to gain admission to a medical school, and then to pass tests with enough or more margin to be awarded the M.D. degree. Having invested so heavily to this end, they come to their house-staff training relatively open to influence.

Since the Flexner report and the changes that followed it some of the gross differences and inadequacies of medical schools have been corrected; the layman is no longer exposed to doctors whose "training" may have consisted of the purchase of a diploma.[2] Now we accept relatively high standards in medical schools as basic, and concern ourselves with improvements and refinements beyond the newly attained standard. But success and improvement here as elsewhere stirs self-criticism and efforts toward more improvement.[3] Recent work of social scientists promises to add a perspective to ongoing efforts of medical educators toward upgrading education beyond medical school. Clearly, more attention and study must turn toward hospitals as learning environments.[4]

The Coggeshall report for the Association of American Medical Colleges, *Planning for Medical Progress through Education*, emphasizes the need to see medical education as a continuing process rather than as a single attainment. "At present, the M.D. degree is earned at about the mid-point of the formal education of the physician. It is recognized that the doctor is not fully qualified to practice at this point, but it is here that the traditional medical school abandons him and relinquishes responsibility. In the future, professional physician education should continue in a coordinated sequence under the sponsorship and guidance of university medical schools, through internship and residency programs."[5]

For years the medical profession has watched house-staff programs with interest, and has recorded and summarized trends and provided an abundance of material for analysis each year. The Annual Internships and Residencies issues of the *Journal of the American Medical Association* provide detailed breakdowns, by hospitals, of specifics for doctors and students to use when they differentiate between the various internship positions offered. Medical students, educators, hospital administrators, and others are directed, by the selection of statistics and facts, to make comparisons along these dimensions. The *Journal's* tables imply that variables such as number of beds, hospital affiliation, autopsy rate, and number of house-staff positions are worth weighing as possible indicators of the nature of experience the trainee is likely to meet in different hospitals. Social scientists only recently have started to attend to what doctors have known for some time—that the internship and residency experience is widely varied and that some of the variations are significant in the development of the physician.[6]

As Samuel Bloom observed, "There is much reason to believe that the internship and residency contribute more to the socialization of the professional than any other experiences. This is the crucial period when the values to which the individual has been exposed in the medical school and the hospital are most likely to find their final internalized form and become the basis upon which the new physician begins to make decisions for himself."[7] Leland McKittrick points to the significance of internship and residency from the perspective of the medical educator: "As noted by the commission, formal education in preparation for practice is now about equally divided between the time spent in medical school and that spent in training for whatever specialty the young physician may elect. I am in agreement with the many who feel that the intern and resident years may be and probably are the most important of the physician's educational career. Never before has education at this level been studied carefully."[8]

In the early summer of 1958, I worked as a research assistant at Columbia University's Bureau of Applied Social Research. A nationwide study of internships and residencies was planned to provide material on the organizational context, and on interns and residents themselves, in a stratified random sample of hospitals. Its purpose was "to investigate characteristics of the learning process that interns and residents undergo, and to identify some of the factors that are relevant to this learning process."[9] The study also included follow-up material on the interns and residents who had previously been part of the Bureau's panel studies of medical students in four medical schools.

As part of the exploratory field work, I undertook a qualitative study of two hospitals. The two hospitals were similar. Each offered intern positions through the National Internship Matching Plan; each had residency training programs in more than one specialty approved by the Council on Medical Education and Hospitals of the American Medical Association. Both hospitals also enjoyed reputations for excellence in their own community. But these two hospitals also provided some obvious contrasts and thus offered promise for a comparative exploration of the possible impact of selected differences that might "make a difference" in the professional life of the developing physician.

The first hospital, the one called University Hospital in this book, had 1,200 beds. The second, Community Hospital, had fewer than 400 beds. The hospitals were different in other ways: the first was closely affiliated with a medical school and the other was not; the first was in the heart of a major metropolis, the second was located in a town about forty-five miles from the metropolis. I devoted several months to data collection through field observation and interviewing in each hospital—University

Hospital in 1958–1959, and Community Hospital in middle and late 1959.

During 1961 and 1962, I returned to these two hospitals for observation of the period around the first of July when one year's house-staff members are replaced by another. I learned early in the course of work at University Hospital that nearly every significant pattern and theme that characterized the environment and its house-staff program was forecast in my field notes—both in observations and interviews with new interns —on the first day of internship.[10]

An early draft of the report was sent to each of the two hospitals in the study in the hope that any glaring errors in perception or recording or perspective might be detected, or any bias challenged. The administrator of Community Hospital read it and circulated the draft within his hospital. At University Hospital, a full-time attending physician read the report, as well as a sociologist in the hospital and a part-time attending physician. Suggestions that came from these circulated drafts were used in revising subsequent drafts. They were of great benefit, and supportive comments of those who read the report, and who had made study in these hospitals a pleasure, encouraged me to pursue some themes.

In 1962 I interviewed physicians in one southern community around the issues of relationship between town and gown in medicine.[11] About half the interviews were with full-time professors in a hospital associated with a medical school. The rest were with local practitioners who had admitting privileges at a hospital similar in a number of attributes to Community Hospital of this study. These interviews with physicians who had completed their training and were then actively concerned with the relationship between local practitioners and professors who worked *only* within the medical-school hospital offered an opportunity to investigate from another source and perspective some implications of different orientations.

In the ten years since my first concentrated work in the two hospitals, I have observed and interviewed house-staff members, nurses, aides, social workers, attending physicians, and administrators in some sixteen other hospitals throughout the country. As a medical sociologist I have worked with residents, attending physicians, nurses, and social workers in three more hospitals.

In 1968, with the assistance of the Commonwealth Fund and the encouragement and help of Dean Robert Ebert of Harvard Medical School, I was able to visit five different hospitals within one midwestern community. The five hospitals accounted for all but one of the 125 American-trained interns who came to the city's hospitals in one year. Programs in these hospitals were approved by the Councils on Medical Education and on Hospitals of the American Medical Association. The five hospitals presented an array of some of the distinctly different kinds of hospitals that train most interns today. In two hospitals I was able to observe and interview at the end of internship year and then again as the new group arrived to begin their house-staff year. The fact that the two hospitals held their initiations on different days, the one on the first of July and the other on the Sunday before the first of July, allowed me to study two first days of internship in one year.

As part of the field work for this study I accompanied individual house-staff members on their regular assignments—as they admitted patients, served in the emergency room, did examinations on rounds or during admission work, worked in the laboratory, discussed patients, studied X-rays, and chatted over coffee-breaks with other doctors, nurses, social workers, and administrators.

During many observation periods, I was able to ask questions and conduct brief supplementary interviews around situations observed, as house-staff members seemed disposed to take a few minutes off between duties to chat. Some of the situational "interviews" took place as the observer and an intern or resident walked along corridors or sat in the nursing station, or in a hospitality shop or treatment room. These frequent occasions for brief questions *in situ* provided opportunities to ask the person observed about an experience or situation while the event was fresh in the minds of both respondent and interviewer.[12] Such occasions also offered chances to correct some misconceptions and to explore matters that had been—and might otherwise have remained—overlooked in more formal interviews. At times a question about an event of which both respondent and interviewer shared first-hand knowledge led the intern or resident to muse about attributes of the environment as he experienced them. Frequently, observations and explanations house-staff members volunteered in these on-the-spot situations suggested that physicians-in-training sometimes liked to take on the role of a consultant for the field work. When they did so, they almost always opened up new areas the observer could investigate, or added comprehension in areas already open.

Attending physicians, directors of nurses, chiefs of services, chief pharmacists, pathologists in charge of laboratories, social workers in several positions, head nurses, and a few hospital volunteers were also subjects for focused interviews of an hour and more. Additional information offered during subsequent informal chats supplemented most of the interviews.

Organizational material and data were obtained through records and reports from the record librarian, director of voluntary services, hospital administration, and social workers of each hospital. Records and printed material from each hospital provided some check on impressions from observations and interviews, and at the same time, opened new approaches toward understanding relationships between different parts of the environment and between members in these two hospitals. In addition to the field work and interviews, data for this study were collected through a survey of house-staff members.

A questionnaire designed as part of a nationwide survey of interns and residents was sent by the Bureau of Applied Social Research to all American-trained interns and residents on four major services (medicine, surgery, obstetrics-gynecology, and pediatrics) of 167 hospitals that were a stratified random sample of hospitals with approved training programs. A 64 percent response gave us 3,297 usable questionnaires. Results from this nationwide survey provide quantitative checks on qualitative observations, and results from the survey are offered where they relate to themes of this report.

A similar questionnaire was mailed to 72 of University Hospital's 195 house-staff members and 9 American-trained interns at Community Hospital. Written-in comments on these questionnaires offered valuable elaboration of, and clues to the meaning that individual respondents attached to questions.[13]

My clearance for work on individual services of the two study hospitals came primarily through different channels and offered an early example of differences in the patterns of interaction, access to information, and also authority relationships in the two environments. At University Hospital a full-time attending physician and professor in the affiliated medical school, who was the medical consultant for the larger study, gained acceptance for the study through chiefs of services. These physicians—full time in their hospital—were key figures whose auspices provided not only permission to observe and interview but also invaluable acceptability by the house-staff members on their services.[14]

For entry into Community Hospital, the medical consultant for the larger Internship-Residency study called a physician he knew on the Community Hospital attending staff. The man at Community Hospital was chief of a service and director of education. He accepted the idea of observation in his hospital and suggested I call the hospital administrator for an appointment. With the initial approval from the one chief of service, the administrator and his secretary at Community Hospital gave me permission to interview and observe house staff and attending physicians alike, somewhat as individual chiefs of services did at University Hospital.[15] At Community Hospital the administrator introduced me to key people—the pharmacist, director of nurses, the head of volunteers. Then the director of nurses invited me to one of her staff meetings and introduced me as a sociologist who "will be with us for a while." I was thus helped into the setting of Community Hospital by a series of personal introductions to all the people I would be seeing—a forecast of the social climate of the hospital.

Modern general hospitals of at least 300 beds, and with approved training programs, offer some advantages for study by participant observation. Many people in different statuses routinely move about the floors and into patients' rooms. These workers are often accepted without much question by virtue of their status, whether or not they are known personally. They are often identified by a uniform, and in this context, the white "lab coat" of the observer provides a kind of acceptability that arouses little curiosity among patients and workers. Once a few key people knew I would be working in their area, and accepted the work as legitimate, my introduction into the setting seldom stimulated comment or question.[16] Rose Coser also reports that the new person on a ward in a teaching hospital is readily accepted as long as he wears a white coat.[17]

A hospital presents a good environment for observation because of the nature of work done there. When house-staff members worked together over a critically ill patient or discussed a diagnosis, their attention was often so fully captured by urgent problems that they had little thought for self-consciously altering their behavior and words for the benefit of an observer. Kenneth Clute reports repeated instances where doctors said the correct thing and then did the opposite. Clute suggests, however, that the doctor's behavior was probably little influenced over sustained periods of observations. Some practitioners, during the first hour or two of the visit, were probably doing things they did not usually do. But they seemed rather quickly to revert to their habitual patterns under pressure of time.[18] House-staff members at University Hospital were used to working with a high degree of visibility. They spend much time working in teams and with various physicians "looking over their shoulder." Some of them were even accustomed to being investigated by sociologists, and reported they had already answered many questions in our studies of medical students. They were generally less self-conscious about being observed than were the Community Hospital interns. One intern from Community Hospital reported later that he had at first found it difficult to have someone follow him around. In another nonaffiliated hospital on July 1, an administrator introduced an intern to me, explaining that I would be with the intern through the day. The new arrival accepted this added burden for a stressful day with poise. But there was an understandable moment of hesitation, and the question, "For how long will you be following me?"

Within each hospital the good will and intelligent interest of many people were an essential aid in my work. The professional commitment of people in hospitals to "help" and their commitments to investigate and search for ways to improve programs and health care contribute a degree of acceptability to hospital observation that many field workers in hospitals seem to enjoy today—an acceptability that is not so abundantly available in other contexts.

A number of William Foote Whyte's recommendations about field work are still particularly appropriate for studying hospitals today.[19] First among them is his recommendation to keep key people informed about the moves of the field worker. This can reassure people in the host organization that the observer is responsibly in touch with organizational channels. At the same time the contacts provide regular chances for key people to volunteer information and perspectives, and the contact can also provide an "early warning system" against potentially disruptive definitions of the field work.[20]

Whyte also cautioned the observer to conform to the standards of behavior of the people under observation, and to offer simple explanations of purpose for the study. Traditional medical standards for protection of patients and their privacy add reasons why the observer in a hospital must be meticulous about confidential information and must resist any temptation to relay seemingly innocuous remarks or "gossip."

The observer is obliged to attend consciously to defining his role for the people he will observe. If he does not, he can find that people around him have elaborated their own definitions and this can have unfortunate results.[21] Upon first arriving on a ward, unless it seemed intrusive at the time I told the nurses and physicians in charge that I was "studying internships and residencies in hospitals."[22] After that I attempted to work in one area for at least a few days so people there would get used to me.[23] I made no attempt to conceal the fact of observation and recording. My decision to be somewhat more open about observing and recording than some observers suggest was based in part on an impression of the particular organization—and the guess that it would not seem intrusive there. I was also influenced by my own quite subjective discomfort about concealment. Peter Blau adds still another argument on behalf of candor. "The feelings of insecurity that the bureaucratic field situation tends to evoke in the observer . . . are generally a major source of blunders. This is the fundamental pragmatic reason, quite aside from considerations of professional ethics, why the observer, in my opinion, should not resort to concealment and deception."[24]

As William Goode and Paul Hatt note, "Purely nonparticipant observation is difficult. We have no standard set of relationships or role patterns for the nonmember who is always present, but never participating. Both the group and the outsider are likely to feel uncomfortable."[25] In a hospital context where many people are often very active and busy, and where some medical workers do occasionally take notes in the course of their work, note-taking by the observer conforms to behavior patterns of numerous workers. I used shorthand and there were moments when note-taking provided me with visible, but not unusual, work. At times it would have been even more difficult to stand by, with no apparent function to perform, in the face of fear and death or pain. I sometimes felt protected by being able to take notes, and in some situations my field reports, dictated from voluminous shorthand notes, included material that I would otherwise have forgotten, either because it was anxiety-provoking or because it did not fit neatly into a preconception I had held.[26] Use of shorthand notes and immediate dictation to tape, I believe, helped me avoid some loss and bias through selective attention, perception, and recall. I took pains to separate my objective observations from my hunches and ideas by setting all these interpretations off with parentheses in my field reports.[27]

My consistent recording of what people said seemed to encourage some to add comments or discussion. Occasionally, interns or residents and others volunteered their interpretation or evaluation of an event or situation in a way that suggested it was reassuring to have someone so interested in all they thought about their work, and what they said and did. On a few occasions when someone did comment, "Don't take this down, but . . .," I did, of course, abide by the request. At times I think I bene- fited from being clearly identified as someone from the outside (but with a "legitimate" purpose)—the "stranger" to whom some were willing to be quite candid about their current problems.[28]

Focused interviews provided occasions to pursue private def- initions behind comments and actions and to ask individuals what they thought had influenced their opinions, what aspects of work they valued, and what they felt they could disregard. Many respondents were articulate and introspective, so that in- terviews were often most productive and contributed toward development of hypotheses about the impact of specific aspects of house-staff experience.[29]

The two hospitals presented in this study have been used to facilitate analysis following Weber's use of "ideal types."[30] Neither hospital is ideal in the sense of being perfect, nor aver- age in the statistical sense. As with any typology, these descrip- tions accentuate significant differences by specifying discrete observations and facts and presenting them in an analytical construct. The two first days did progress as I described them in two hospitals. As with any thematic analysis, many comments, exchanges, and gestures have been left out—either because they seemed irrelevant for analysis or because they were apparently unique to the one hospital. In the course of observing and in- terviewing on other initiation days and in other hospitals, I have been able to compare and select so that these descriptions convey something of the essence of consequential differences between hospitals. Julien Freund's comments on the use of typologies is appropriate: ". . . because the mind is not capable of reproducing or copying reality, but only of reconstructing it with the aid of concepts. And there is an infinite distance between the real and the conceptual . . . whatever method we use, we can only impose an order of relationships on reality, not exhaust it."[31]

Hospitals within the types I have described in detail are each distinctly individual. I do not assume—nor should the reader—

that every university hospital is like the University Hospital of this study. Also, each community hospital has characteristics of its own and may show some attributes of both the Community and University Hospital of this study. All community hospitals may look alike to a few educators in major teaching centers—though these same men describe in telling detail how very different each university hospital is from every other. But on the other side, some physicians in community hospitals see fine distinctions between their own hospital and other nonaffiliated hospitals they know.

It is time to look at specific aspects within the wide spectrum of hospitals to see how different patterns, values, norms, and attitudes are systematically reinforced, beginning with the first day of internship.

Some of the attributes of social structure and climate found in these two hospitals occur in a variety of other hospitals and with similar effect. It is not size or degree of affiliation, but more specific patterns that come to be associated with these gross attributes that have implications for the profession, medical science, and for the delivery of health care.

I | Trends in Medical Practice and Training

In the 1830's Alexis de Tocqueville commented, "In America the passion for physical well-being is general."[1] Our commitments to change and improvement, to search for a better way to accomplish almost everything, do stimulate interest in medical advances, and our passion for health is supported. The 1970's may see health become the country's principal business. Wider ranges of medical service are provided under the aegis of the hospital, and more of the cost of such services is paid by insurance, group plans, and government subsidy.[2]

Accelerating the search for health today, many people have the leisure and discretionary income to seek improved health and appearance, longevity, relief from discomfort, sleeplessness, or sleepiness.[3] Mass magazines stimulate hope with news of "breakthroughs," sometimes in advance of sufficient research. Politicians and social critics can gain wide publicity by either decrying the use of people in research, or by pointing to the failure of medicine to find a cure for the common cold. Weekly and monthly articles appear with titles like, "The Doctor's Image Is Sickly." Popular books and reports feed ambivalence, discontent or outright distrust of physicians.[4]

Unquestionably, there is room for improvement in many aspects of medical care and delivery of health services. But at the same time there is an element of the unreasonable in some public criticisms. The public demands that it be satisfied, but in the nature of unlimited expectations for improvement complete satisfaction is impossible. Not only are the expectations unlimited, they are also sometimes contradictory. The public does call for more research breakthroughs at the same time it decries the physician's attention to the research implications of a case. The public demands that the physician hold stubbornly to hope and efforts to save life even in the face of great odds. But at the same time it may condemn "heartless measures and indignities" used to keep the patient alive.

The acceleration of progress in medical science and improvements in medical care do not guarantee the medical profession either widespread public gratitude or trust. The public and the individual have high hopes and urgent needs of perfection, if not of miracles, from the medical profession. But at the same time, the public reads of "shameful conditions in hospitals." A patient may live long enough to be disillusioned about an individual hospital and its doctors and nurses. Moreover, medical-scientific progress does not assure the adequate delivery of health care to all segments of the population. Thus, great expectations can throw the spotlight on real deficiencies, and at the same time generate ambivalence.

Sociological ambivalence, a socially induced tendency to be both attracted to and repelled by, to need and at the same time to fear the services of a group, characterizes attitudes toward the medical profession. The professional is thus exposed to ambivalence not only because of his unique personality, but because ambivalence is inherent in the situation he occupies. "In the anxious eyes of the client virtually every remark and act of the professional are imbued with disproportionate significance . . . All this tends to produce an excess of emotional response: exaggerated praise . . . and exaggerated blame; . . . emotions . . . become focused on the professional and, by generalization, on the profession at large."[5]

Yet in the face of occasional objective inadequacies and the subjective problems of ambivalence, many individual patients are grateful, trusting, and loyal to their individual physicians. They have to be if they are to allow the professional to help them. The individual patient may handle the stressful problem of ambivalence by believing that his own particular physician of the moment is good and informed and wise, but the profession is bungling, greedy, and unconcerned. The patient can thus muster the necessary trust and still give vent to anger in the face of dependency problems, fearful realities, limits, and anxieties. At least one survey has found that ambivalence toward physicians generally appears to be a characteristic attitude of the people who accord physicians the highest prestige.[6]

Anger against the physician is, of course, not new. In the fifteenth century, Pope John XXII burned an unsuccessful physician in Florence, and when John himself died, his friends flayed the surgeon who had failed to keep the prelate alive.[7] Although present-day feelings may not be new, our ways of expressing them are somewhat different.

Some malpractice litigation and large judgments may signify the extent to which laymen hold exaggerated notions of what can and should come from medical efforts. A bad result at times seems to be taken as almost necessarily implying criminal lack of skill, or negligence.[8] Along with this, however, there is also the reality of shocking neglect and shabby medical performance by some practitioners and in some hospitals. Repeated suits against a few suggest that something more objective than ambivalence can also cause litigation.

As more people turn more readily to the hospital and are more knowledgeable about and demanding of good medical care, their criticisms of medicine are likely to become more salient. Outpatient departments become more crowded and more people object. Regular visits to these departments increased 30 percent in a recent four-year period, and emergency visits increased 81 percent. Related to the shift of care toward hospitals, more physicians of many ranks work full time in hospitals, and the trend continues. Full-time medical school clinical faculty, for example, grew from 2,276 in 1951 to more than 10,000 in 1965. The number is predicted to reach 19,000 by 1975. Milton Roemer estimated that 35 percent of the nation's doctors in 1966 were on full-time salary and another third of them held part-time appointments.[9]

The other side of this increase in the number of salaried positions in medicine is a decline both in the number of physicians in solo practice and a further reduction of the ranks of physi-

cians in general practice.[10] Thus there are fewer physicians willing to make house calls, and fewer physicians who will care for
a single family for a lifetime. Moreover, the move of physicians
away from isolated offices exposes more of the doctor's work to
potential scrutiny. Table 1 shows the trend toward diminution

TABLE 1
FAMILY PHYSICIAN POTENTIAL (M.D.), SELECTED YEARS

Type of private practice	1931	1940	1949	1957	1965
Pediatrics	1,396	2,222	3,787	5,876	9,726
Internal medicine	3,567	5,892	10,923	14,654	22,432
General practice	112,116	109,272	95,526	81,443	65,951
Total	117,079	117,386	110,236	101,973	98,109
Total per 100,000 population	94	89	75	60	50

Source: Rashi Fein, *The Doctor Shortage: An Economic Diagnosis* (Washington,
D.C.: The Brookings Institute, 1967), Table III-4, p. 72.

of the ranks of physicians who served as primary or family physicians of several decades ago. Lyden, Geiger, and Peterson's survey compared physicians who were graduated from medical
school in 1950 with those from the class of 1954.[11] The portion
of medical school graduates who listed their present field of
practice as general practice declined, and the percentage of those
in teaching and research went up. By 1967 just 23 percent of all
physicians were still in general practice. But the trainees on duty
in this field represented less than one percent of all men in general practice and only 1.5 percent of all trainees on duty.[12]

Graduate Education of Physicians

Medical education, too, has not escaped public attention. Here
also, the actual situation has improved since the turn of the century. Major reforms followed the 1910 Flexner report, and the
subsequent implementation of recommendations came through
the Council on Medical Education of the American Medical Association and the Association of American Medical Colleges.
At that time many promising and dedicated young men of this
country were traveling to Europe for medical education and
post-graduate work. Today the direction of migration for "the

best and most advanced" has nearly reversed. Many promising European physicians today seek residency training or training fellowship in American hospitals and universities.[13]

Part of the present strength of medical education stems from the fact that our contemporary medical schools include elements of the two European types that Flexner described. The clinical type native to France and Great Britain was concentrated in the hospital so that the student was not so much a student of the university as a disciple or apprentice to the clinician. That system produced some great clinicians. In contrast, the university type tended to separate the student from bedside experience. The renowned researcher taught in Germany, Scandinavia, Holland, and German-speaking Switzerland. Under this system medical theory and research prospered and specialization and differentiation developed most rapidly. The present three-way association between hospital, university, and research laboratory is rather new to the history of medicine and this new arrangement is significant for both advancing techniques of diagnosis and treatment and stimulating innovation in hospitals.

As with improvements in medical science, improvements in medical education will not assure public accolades. Quite the opposite. With expectations raised, new benchmarks are set. High training standards in medical school and the extension of training and improvements in the house-staff programs are a part of what the public accepts as given. From there it will continue to expect improvements at an accelerated rate. It is precisely the improvements that raise expectations and then frustrations.

Many medical students—only yesterday a part of the lay public—are articulate, insistent, and convey a sense of mission as they challenge the profession and medical education. Chants of "Hip, Hip Hippocrates, Up with Service, Down with Fees," rock the decorum of formal medical meetings. Medical schools add students to curriculum and other committees in efforts to keep up with the demands, but demands continue to increase. Many of these dedicated recruits to medicine promise much for future health, though as with some medical procedures, not without some pain in the process of therapy.

Change is inevitable and so is continued criticism. If the educator were to set out to produce programs and men to satisfy the public on all counts all the time, he would be destined to frustration. But in view of some of the urgency of demands and the visibility of medical matters—and accepting the positive contribution that a restless and demanding public makes toward stimulating search for improvements—awareness of the difference in lay and medical perspectives and attention to the laymen's demands seems essential.

Social Functions of the Medical Profession

It is characteristic of a profession that its members believe that their work is special and worthy of note and esteem, and that laymen also accord it prestige. Professionals share a collective identity with those who have gone through similar training, as well as attachment to the work itself. The extended training that professions typically demand develops the sense of identity that is indispensable if members are to care about what happens to their profession. With this, the profession can fulfill some of its social functions. It can control its members through pressures and sanctions not available to the layman, who is hardly able to judge performance. It has the strength to protect its members from excessive visibility and judgment about matters that the layman cannot understand and where lay evaluations may be faulty. It can set standards of training and performance and seek to improve them; and it can improve itself also through recruitment and training.

It would be unwise to expect patients, who are generally at some distance from medical science, to make knowledgeable distinctions about the way some medical problems are handled. Medical prohibitions such as those against advertising help protect patients against a choice of medical help that would be based on nonrelevant information.

Physicians since Hippocrates have noted with varying degrees of dismay that lay evaluations of the physician are often based on interpersonal skills, extraneous symbols, or purported "cures," and do not always coincide with the evaluations by physicians. In the ambiguous and anxiety-provoking situation the patient faces when he is not well, he often looks for clues he *can* understand: how "interested" in him the physician seems to be, the physician's manner, and secondary characteristics such as appearance, race, religion, sex, the equipment he sees, or the way the office looks. The patient comes with needs for absolute cure and reassurance, yet the physician has to be aware of uncertainty in diagnosis and treatment, and he must often work with probability, not certitude.[14]

The physician is supposed to judge medical qualifications on the bases of extent of medical information and acumen, and length and quality of training. The profession evaluates willingness to share information or admit limits to knowledge, willingness to abide by the profession's standards, thoroughness in medical history-taking and care in diagnosis and planning for therapy. The layman may take less note of these matters than he does of the way the doctor talks to him, or how well he feels after seeing a doctor.[15] One physician, discussing training programs, observed: "I can look back on a number of occasions when I learned to my surprise that an intern whom I considered to be the less able member of his group was regarded by many of the patients to be the one indispensable member of the staff."[16] An attending physician at Community Hospital commented that a physician "could be thoroughly detested" by physicians and still "make a living in the community." The often cited Osler Peterson survey of medical practice in North Carolina found little association between excellence of work (as judged by visiting medical colleagues) and lay approval (as implied by income of the physician).[17]

Dr. Oliver Wendell Holmes wrote about the gap between laymen's and physicians' bases for medical judgments:

> In the first place, the persons who seek the aid of the physician are very honest and sincere in their wish to get rid of their complaints, and generally speaking, to live as long as they can . . . There is nothing men will not do, there is nothing they have not done, to recover their health and save their lives. They have submitted to be half-drowned in water, and half-cooked with gases, to be buried up to their chins in earth, to be seared with hot irons like galley-

slaves, to be crimped with knives, like codfish, to have needles thrust into their flesh, and bonfires kindled on their skin, to swallow all sorts of abominations, and to pay for all this, as if to be singed and scalded were a costly privilege, as if blisters were a blessing, and leeches were a luxury. What more can be asked to prove their honesty and sincerity? This same community is very intelligent with respect to a great many subjects—commerce, mechanics, manufactures, politics. But with regard to medicine it is hopelessly ignorant and never finds it out.[18]

Professional people sometimes use the terms *quack, charlatan, popularizer,* or *shyster,* to convey their distaste for a fellow professional "gone wrong," for one who responds to hopes and rewards of some laymen so much that he deviates far from *professional* norms. The quack and charlatan promise cures that patients demand, the popularizer may receive acclaim in mass magazines, the shyster over-responds to a client's demands to win his case. Such catering to the public in itself does violence to the professional ethic. It denies the professional spirit of being at one with colleagues. It competes unfairly against them.[19] On the other side, the layman uses terms such as *callous* or *cold* to express his resentment when the professional fails to live up to lay expectations. The physician does not do the "kind" thing, but orders a painful diagnostic procedure and so "doesn't care" for his patient.

To remedy this situation, it is sometimes assumed that more and better communication is both possible and productive.[20] However, some distance between laymen and physician can be at times useful for both. David Riesman speculates that a client approaching his lawyer is in a sense protected by the "mystery" of the law. He can thus throw virtually the whole burden on his counsel. The lawyer, unaware of the psychological roots of this division of labor, may at times try in vain to "educate" his client.[21] Similarly, physicians who strive to educate patients toward facing uncertainties of treatment also struggle with the difficulty that patients want to be protected, at least in some measure, from the insecurities which dampen their hopes.

Some air of mystery about work may also protect the professional so that he can perform successfully.[22] At one extreme, when there is too little distance between patient and physician when the physician is too dependent on the patient's approval, that physician may escape from control of his medical colleagues. Some important goals of scientific medicine will suffer, and so will patients, as when the physician overattends to conveying the *impression* of interest, the *impression* of careful diagnosis and certainty, or when he loses some necessary degree of objectivity. At the other extreme, the physician can become so preoccupied with approval of the medical-scientific community that his patients are left unduly frightened, unduly tested and inconvenienced, and his practice-oriented medical colleagues out in the community are left bewildered and resentful.

Physicians who receive their training in a value climate that places relatively more emphasis on action, flexibility, and on establishing rapport may develop skills and techniques for dealing with patients and for putting knowledge into practice with dispatch. However, "interest" in the patient beyond a certain point may interfere with effective treatment and judgment.[23] Also, rewards enjoyed for facility with action and for rapport with patients can lead the practitioner beyond the limits of his knowledge.

Division of Function in the Network of Hospitals

The programs in closely affiliated hospitals provide good chances that physicians will be identified with their specialty and its associations. Men in these programs are likely to establish strong bonds with colleagues within a specialty and become committed to medical-scientific norms. These men, often working with groups of physicians, may be somewhat insulated from lay demands, and at times may seem to be unresponsive to patients. The climate and structure of some university hospitals attracts and then encourages physicians who are committed to the norms governing medical research.

Nonaffiliated hospitals do not offer their physicians-in-training these mutually reinforcing conditions of specialty identification in such abundance. They offer more chances for identifying with some other norms, such as interest in the patient's response and the patient's family situation. Should the community hospitals of the country receive effective support for residency programs—for example, the type of extended training for the "primary physician" recommended in the Millis report —they could offer the prolonged stay that seems a prerequisite for identification within the house-staff group.[24] Relegating the community hospitals to a more isolated position in the medical-education enterprise reduces the chances for effective social control of these physicians who are pushed out to the fringes of the profession. Effective consultation and continuing education of the private practitioners are also likely to suffer.

Only 138 of the 7,000 hospitals in the country have more than 500 beds, a major university affiliation, and an approved internship program. Their number is increasing as new medical schools are opened.[25] But what happens within the ranks of the full-time medical educators and the major teaching centers that develop and sustain them is more significant and has more impact than even their expanding numbers would indicate.

Although some of these hospitals are quite large, together they provide only 8 percent of the nation's hospital beds. But in one year this small number of hospitals was able to attract over 45 percent of all nonforeign interns.[26] Advances in medical

TABLE 2
RELATION OF HOSPITAL AFFILIATION TO U.S. HOSPITAL BEDS

	Hospitals		Hospital beds	
	Number of hospitals	% of total	Number of beds	% of total
Hospitals with approved programs				
Major medical school affiliation	339	4	165,550	10
Limited medical school affiliation	147	2	94,408	6
Graduate medical school affiliation	121	2	44,526	2
No medical school affiliation	905	12	474,980	28
Totals	1,512	21	779,464	46
Hospitals without approved training programs	5,658	79	899,194	54
Grand totals (American Hospital Association)	7,160	100	1,678,658	100

Source: American Medical Association, *Directory of Approved Internships and Residencies* (1967), p. 17.

science and research and some advances in delivery of health care are largely products of such hospital centers. Table 2 summarizes the relation of hospital affiliation to hospital beds.

Patient admission patterns in some of the nonmetropolitan affiliated hospitals exemplify an extreme in specialized function in the country's complex of medical training, research, diagnosis, treatment, and care. The University Hospital of this study, for example, screens patients before admitting them, selecting them along criteria of potential as teaching material, as candidates for one of the many research projects, and the patient's need for hospitalization in the specialized center. Residents explain that there are other hospitals in the community to which patients can be referred. Without some purposive limits to admission at University Hospital, patients who have specific needs for its elaborate diagnostic and treatment facilities might not be able to gain admission at the time when they need it.

Deep in the medical academic world, a physician may rarely see a patient except in the presence of other physicians. As we shall see, this pattern helps to protect the medical-school culture and its commitments to advancing knowledge and scientific excellence. But at the same time there can also be some unfortunate consequences in a university hospital from the "committee" care of patients.[27]

A second and quite distinct culture weaves medicine into the world of laymen through thousands of local unaffiliated hospitals and the private practices around them. Thus, a few hospitals do most of the training of American-trained physicians and turn out most of the research, as well as the academic physicians who will influence the development of future physicians. But the largest number of hospitals in the country, the ones that provide most of the hospital beds, have little or no direct contact with what happens in the academic centers. The community hospitals get the slimmest portions of research and training grants. In one year, less than one percent of all separate (National Institutes of Health) grants of all sizes found their way into the small unaffiliated hospitals.[28] These hospitals are relatively far removed from the planning and decisions that affect distribution of manpower, funds, and curriculum time in medical schools and from the over-all planning about the medical care system. But these nonaffiliated hospitals are in a position to have much influence on the practice of medicine in local communities. Their orientation, interests, and support tend to be concentrated within their local communities. When many laymen think of hospitals, it is their own community hospital which serves as their prototype.

Internationally, the university and the community hospitals of the country also seem to provide differently for health care, present and future. The large research and teaching centers make major contributions to the science of medicine in the world. Foreign scientists visit these centers when they come to this country, and they follow research reports that come from these institutions. Community hospitals train large numbers of foreign graduates, many of whom return to provide health care in their native lands. Providing the nation with 28 percent of its hospital beds, these affiliated, community hospitals offer about 44 percent of all approved internships. But this is a problem because many of these internship positions go unfilled and many more are occupied by graduates of foreign medical schools that represent various degrees of training standards and experience.[29]

Recruitment to nonaffiliated hospitals, like recruitment into general practice, is losing ground (see Fig. 1). The proportion of nonaffiliated hospitals receiving more than one half of the interns they sought through the matching plan fell from 31 percent in 1958 to 23 percent in 1968. Of the 193 hospitals with major medical school affiliations, 149 or 77 percent received over half of their interns through the National Intern Matching Program.[30]

Community hospitals developed as teaching centers in the post-World War II period, the time when returning medical officers sought graduate training in specialties and there were too few programs and residency positions to meet the need. By the Korean War, the trend had turned and there were beginning to be too many positions and too few residents. The non-affiliated community hospitals were hardest hit. Among efforts to upgrade educational programs, a new position, "Director of

Fig. 1. Percentage of NIMP participants matched to major affiliated hospitals, minor affiliated hospitals, and nonaffiliated hospitals, 1952–1967.

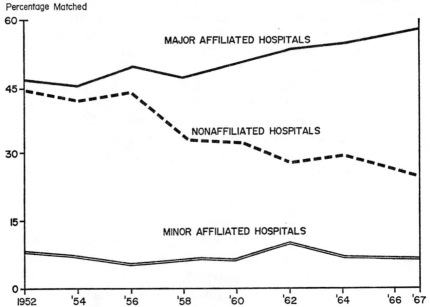

Percentage Matched

MAJOR AFFILIATED HOSPITALS

NONAFFILIATED HOSPITALS

MINOR AFFILIATED HOSPITALS

60
45
30
15
0

1952   '54   '56   '58   '60   '62   '64   '66 '67

Source: Division of Operational Studies, "Results of the National Intern Matching Program for 1967," *Journal of Medical Education*, 42 (1967), 626.

Medical Education," was added to many programs. By 1965 there were 970 of these directors, over half of them full time and on salary, in community hospitals.[31] But the nonaffiliated hospitals still have a more difficult time attracting American-trained house-staff members.

The recent recruitment results of several hospitals I visited within one midwestern community conveys some trends. Thirteen hospitals in the community have internship training programs approved by the Council on Medical Education and Hospitals of the American Medical Association. In 1966 there were 232 internship positions offered. Of these, 125 were filled by nonforeign students, 72 went unfilled, and foreign graduates filled the remaining positions.

The midwestern city that I visited is the home of a widely respected university with a medical school, and two of the city's hospitals are affiliated with it. They only accepted two of all the foreign interns in the city that year. Together, these two affiliated hospitals accounted for a third of the approved internship positions available in the city, and they recruited 58 percent of all the American-trained interns. A single nonaffiliated hospital accounted for another 22 percent of all nonforeign interns in approved positions; a second one added 17 percent. But all nine of the other community hospitals together had attracted less than 3 percent of all the American-trained interns in the city, although they had 44 percent of all the city's approved positions.[32]

Figure 2 summarizes sixteen years of internship placement in this community. Hospitals A and B are the ones with medical school affiliations. They have shown a fairly consistent ability to recruit interns through the National Intern Matching Plan, and they attract more of the American-trained medical students now than they did ten and fifteen years ago. In contrast, all but one

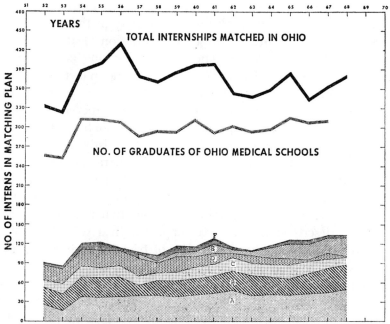

Fig. 2. Recruitment of American-trained interns in Ohio, 1951-1968.

of the nonaffiliated hospitals (C, D, and F) show some decline in the number of American-trained interns they attract. One of these hospitals also shows some marked fluctuation in the results of recruiting efforts—a pattern to be discussed later, for it is not unusual in community hospitals. Only one of the hospitals without university affiliation (Hospital E) has been able to obtain increasing numbers of interns through the matching plan. This hospital is atypical among nonaffiliated hospitals in that all of its attending physicians are full time. It is also unique in its expansive facilities and well-endowed, vigorous education programs for physicians in practice as well as for house-staff members. The ascendancy of medical schools in the network of hospitals is a portent of more change to come in the medical care system. University affiliation is widely accepted as adding to hospital prestige.[33]

Both university affiliation and hospital size are relatively easy to determine, as well as potentially significant, and they are used throughout this book. It should be clear, however, that not every hospital of the same size and degree of affiliation is like University Hospital. There is also infinite variety in the community hospitals of the country. Part of the variation relates to other elements that make a difference in the learning environment that interns and residents will find. For example, the portion of attending physicians who are full time in a hospital can largely influence training experiences. Where supervision is provided by men with a busy practice away from the hospital, the intern's work is less subject to review and less visible. He is more quickly pushed to work alone than he is where there are many full-time people around him. The size of the community in which the hospital serves can also have an impact on the nature of work and life in the hospital. The fact that the Community Hospital described in the next chapter is in a suburban town contributes positively to the quality of friendly exchange in the hospital.

The magnitude as well as the source of major financial support are also important variables that have not been singled out for separate consideration but are acknowledged in this study. The largesse of an extremely wealthy benefactor interested in medical education can powerfully enhance recruiting efforts in a private hospital. As interns sat at lunch on their first day in a well-appointed staff dining room of the nonaffiliated Hospital E, they compared notes on some of the circumstances that had led them to apply to the hospital where they were beginning. Among the major reasons, one intern noted that his specialty interest could be well met in this hospital. Then he added, and his new colleagues agreed, "Also, there is something to be said for practicing medicine in an attractive setting, and I found the other hospital I considered was depressing to me when I went there for an interview." The hospital he came to has a magnificent education building and facilities that are both well planned and beautifully executed.

Variations in the patient populations of hospitals where physicians train can also be important for their learning experiences. House-staff physicians at both Community Hospital and University Hospital see ward and private patients, and in this they have similar problems and experiences, although they handle them differently. There are the clear differences between the experience of treating the public or ward patients compared to treating the private patients within a single hospital. It follows from this that house-staff experience in a city or metropolitan hospital with university affiliation will be distinctly different from experience in a private affiliated setting like University Hospital.

The authority of the physician who is still in training is likely to be a tender attribute—sometimes puffed up and enflamed and subject to hurt when the intern or resident deals with private patients. House-staff members are usually outranked financially by private patients who often do not think of the interns or residents as authorities. Some private patients directly, and others indirectly, indicate they do not need the services of the youthful physician. With the ward patient, the house-staff member, though paid little, can feel he is needed and is offering deserved help. On private duty some interns and residents are jarred into disquieting ideological considerations of their own relatively low financial position compared to that of the patient. Last, and possibly most important, the private patient is not the intern's patient, but the ward patient is. Although the final authority is with the chief resident (or chief of service), the intern is in charge of *his* patient.

In a sense, the exchange of benefits between house staff and ward patient is more even than between the same house-staff member and the private patient on most services. The intern gives service and in return gets to be *the* doctor for the ward patient. The patient provides the chance for learning experience, and sometimes he also agrees to become a research subject in return for the doctor's special interest in him or his medical problem.

A most intangible but vital attribute of the learning environments is the quality of the men and women who are responsible for teaching, supervising, and encouraging the development of excellence in practice, whether that practice is to be in the community, in the medical school, the laboratory, or in a private office. I have seen examples of superb leadership for interns and residents in many different hospitals, and in hospitals oriented toward several different medical directions. The hospital structure and culture can help to attract the superb teacher to lead interns and residents and it can stimulate his best efforts—or subvert them. But without physicians who personify excellence in different types of medical practice the most efficient structure will mean little.

The history of an institution also exerts an influence on the patterns the intern will be exposed to in the hospital. Some hospitals in the United States gained prominence during the time when a hospital was primarily a place of last resort for the indigent sick and for people who had to be kept out of circulation lest they spread infectious diseases. Terms from the past, *fever hospital* and *pesthouse,* and the occasional former juxtaposition of jail and hospital signal this early concept of the hospital. Following the tradition of the hospital as a haven for all applicants, some old and respected centers retain a commitment to admit any patient needing it as a valued part of the hospital ethos. The university-affiliated city hospitals continue this orientation and some of these are able to provide superb care along with commendable training and excellent research.

The propriety of allowing a house-staff member some choice

in screening patients for admission to the ward so that he can select good teaching cases may be most often accepted in the voluntary teaching hospitals that came into prominence in the
1930's and 1940's. Hospitals were then more accepted as the
place of choice for the specialists to diagnose and treat their
middle-class and affluent patients. The most prominent of these
later hospitals were the domains of specialists whose reputations
and names added prestige to the hospital and attracted the most
promising medical graduates for training, as well as the wealthi-
est laymen as benefactors and as patients. Highly trained specialists donated their time and in exchange they often enjoyed
a great deal of autonomy and privilege on their own services.

The house-staff members who worked under these physicians
were paid stipends so small as to be token payment for the service they gave to hospital and patients. But in exchange for long
hours and meager pay, such house-staff members had an opportunity to work under men whose reputations they admired.
Some hoped to become protégés. The prospects of affiliating
with an esteemed hospital tomorrow and excellence of specialty
training today contributed to the motivation to postpone practice on behalf of further training. This pattern also endures in
some respected private hospitals, university-affiliated as well as
unaffiliated.

The house-staff members in such institutions sometimes had
a choice of patients who would be admitted to their teaching
wards. In this system, young physicians began early in their
training to emulate the pattern of the proud specialist-clinician
who saw mostly patients referred by other physicians and who
sometimes selected which patients he would attend. The reputation of the virtuoso physician allowed him a special position in
his hospital. As medicine was practiced, many of the clinician-
teachers in the 1930's and 1940's could also enjoy an aspiring
circle of interns and residents who had competed to be accepted
on their services and who honored brilliance, style, and clinical
acumen. These were social conditions that favored the development of the colorful personality in medicine. Elements of this
pattern remain, but changes in medicine and society have combined to give preeminence to the academic setting and to the

medical team and the house staff rather than to the single successful clinician. More favorable light is being directed to careful investigation and method rather than to the bold diagnostic insight.

House-staff members today are better paid, although not always well paid, and they are given better quarters than formerly. There are more internship and residency positions than there are graduates of American medical schools to fill them. In September 1966 nearly one fourth of all internship positions in the country were unfilled, and even so, graduates of foreign medical schools accounted for 27 percent of the filled positions.[34] House-staff members join together in groups to make demands for better income, housing, and working conditions. More of the interns and residents are married, and they are given more time off than their predecessors. The incoming interns in some teaching hospitals work in a group that wields more influence than interns formerly enjoyed, and they may incline to be somewhat critical of the older men in practice. On the other side, the intern today generally cannot expect either the lavish profits or the singular position to which many former house-staff physicians might have aspired as they watched their chief arrive for rounds.

Community hospitals similar to the one in this study, with approved internship and residency programs and with formal connections to university hospitals through some of their staff members, presently stand somewhere between the two worlds of town and gown. Hence, they are in a good position to help integrate two types of practice which otherwise tend to polarize within the profession. Programs in community hospitals can help to keep alive the possibilities for productive discourse between the men in practice who otherwise are somewhat beyond the influence of the academic centers, and the men in education and research who sometimes are remote from the individual patient and the isolated physician. The community hospitals probably also present wider individual variations than can be found in the large hospitals with major medical-school affiliations. This diversity raises the possibility for the development of hospitals and physicians that can be quickly responsive to the health needs of local communities. If they can function as a point of contact between the two cultures, some programs in the community hospitals may provide evidence for Whitehead's contention: "A clash of doctrines is not a disaster—it is an opportunity."[35] It becomes important first to recognize the fact of different doctrines, different value commitments, different ways of life in medicine, and second, to comprehend how norms, values, and behavior patterns are communicated to each new generation of physicians.

The Social Setting of Internships

Each summer more than eight thousand graduates of American medical schools enter the first year of house-staff training. The first of July, the medical world's formal beginning date for the house-staff year, is a time of dispersion, upheaval, and loss. At the same time it is a period of regrouping, fresh starts, and promise. More than 1,500 hospitals lose a large part of the house-staff they have trained. Yesterday's interns join the ranks of more than 22,000 American-trained residents. In many hospitals a large number of foreign graduates arrive for their first experience in an American hospital, and more move along in residency.[36]

During the time house-staff physicians are changed, a few patients will feel abandoned and some will be frightened at the loss of the young doctors they had come to rely on. Some patients may be discharged a day or two earlier to "clear the wards" in preparation for the arrival of the new staff members. Some patients who are habitués of hospitals or in touch with the grapevine of the community may know that the time just after new house-staff members arrive is the best time to gain admission to crowded space on the wards. The ward, therefore, has its seasonal population changes.

Senior physicians who are active in house-staff training programs can expect that some newcomers will make special demands on their time. The incoming interns may represent the fruit of successful recruiting efforts and the good reputation of the training program. On the other hand, the arrival of only a few nonforeign interns is a reminder to senior staff in some hospitals of the uncertainty of their position in medical education. Hospitals, unable to attract their quota of American-trained interns, may fill out their staff with foreign-trained applicants at some risk to the standing of their training program.

Nurses may feel apprehensive over having a new assortment of young physicians to acquaint with hospital patterns and procedures, or they may welcome the new group as a promising relief from the earlier one with whom they may have had some squabbles. New arrivals can introduce particular stress when the nurse is expected in some ways to lead and instruct doctors who are at this time liable to be especially sensitive to any perceived threat to their new position and authority. In some hospitals, the teaching responsibilities of the nurse are specified in introductions and instructions, and nurses are confirmed as valuable aides to the house staff. In other places very little is said about the function of the nurses in education.

At this same time of change, medical administrators are often forced to alter daily and weekly routines as they bid one year's house-staff members goodbye and welcome new staff. Considerable administrative effort is required to see that necessary keys, instructions, uniforms, living quarters, parking spaces, licenses, physical examinations, insurance, and other details are given adequate attention. Also, administrators and senior physicians must quickly and effectively convey the imperatives of their hospital to the newcomers in order to minimize confusion and risk to patients. The summer vacations of senior physicians add to the stress of those who do stay at work in the hospital during this time.

The coincidence of vacation time for some senior physicians and the introduction of new recruits into the hospital can have unplanned consequences. For example, the newcomer arrives to work at the time when hospitals are possibly more short of staff than they will be later in the year. Thus, in the period when the new house-staff members have most need for supervision there will be the least number of senior physicians available. Under such conditions the house staff may be left to set its own standards and patterns; and these may or may not be the ones that senior-staff members would approve. Possibly, a hasty "hello, welcome, and goodbye" from senior physicians carries a message that negates some of their words about how the patient comes first and how ready everyone in the hospital is to help the newcomer and advise him whenever he needs it.

Hospitals handle this first day of training in many ways. In some places interns are introduced to their new responsibilities a week or a few days early so they can be eased into their assignments before the experienced residents have left or moved up. Some hospitals have a festive breakfast the first day and some have a dinner the night before, with welcoming speeches and introductions. Some hospitals present a detailed program of action to be followed the first day. Some move the intern into his assignment with only a brief greeting over coffee, a packet of instructions, forms, maps, a formulary, and introductions to residents and other interns with whom he will work on his first assignment.* Regardless of these variations, nearly everywhere the arriving interns show signs of apprehension, as well as eagerness to have things go well. Many have moved their families from one area to another with the attendant upset, nuisance, and cost. Some convey uncertainty and confusion during their first hectic days in the hospital; but at the same time, many express great hopes and expectations for the coming year. It might be well in medicine if more of the good intentions and aspirations of many new arrivals could survive the house-staff experience.

Since an article, "The Fate of Idealism in Medical School," appeared ten years ago, much has been written to suggest that as students move through medical school, some of their initial enthusiasm and commitments to ideals of patient care and service lose a bit of their luster. Evidence of this disenchantment, or reduction of enchantment, turns up too often to be ignored. Some change from the perspectives of the layman to a more professional orientation, some realignments between ideal and reality in details may even be necessary to allow for effective functioning.[37]

In the house-staff experience some further attrition of ideals seems to occur as interns and residents cope with the realities

---

* A formulary is a collection of stated and prescribed medicinal preparations approved by the hospital and stocked in its pharmacy.

of their particular hospital. The fresh start implicit in the first day of internship is associated with great expectations. Practically no one enters this phase of a medical career planning to become careless of scientific standards or of treatment. But each hospital throws the spotlight on certain aspects of the intern's work and leaves some work relatively protected against visibility or supervision and thus potentially subject to neglect. In this process each hospital provides selective reinforcement for some ideals and some of the intern's initial commitments, and each hospital allows some leeway around some other ideals. These factors can vary markedly in different learning environments, and they condition which ideals, which standards, and which behavior and professional communication patterns are most consistently reinforced and accepted by the graduate physician.

II | The First of July in Two Hospitals

Internship at University Hospital: Joining a Proud Company

A graduate of one of the country's leading medical schools reported for his first day's duties in a straight medical internship in the 1,200-bed University Hospital, a major medical teaching center.* He had gained his assignment through the National Intern Matching Plan. A professor in his medical school had urged him to take this internship. This was the intern's first choice among the hospitals he considered, and he was one of several of the new interns that people in the hospital had been most eager to recruit.

The hospital he arrived at was built in the 1930's—a tall, imposing block of steel and stone dominating its immediate neighborhood. It is one of seven hospitals in its metropolis having an over 1,000-bed capacity, and it is not the largest among them.

Spacious corridors connect the hospital and the medical school on many levels, and they reflect and reinforce ties between the hospital and its community of medical educators. Just as the network of corridors interpenetrate the medical school and the hospital, other lines connect them in the intern's environment. There are financial ties. Three-budgets—hospital, university,

---

* The straight internship provides training on a surgical, medical, pediatrics, ob-gyn, or pathology service in a hospital holding full approval for a residency program in that specialty. The straight contrasts with mixed internship and with rotating internship where the intern spends a period of time varying from a few weeks to two or more months on each of several services of a hospital.

and a joint budget—allocate financial resources. Salaries for attending physicians who teach represent contributions from both the university and the hospital. Research and library facilities are supported by combinations of funds from these budgets. There are also formal administrative ties; for example, through the joint administrative board of the "University Hospital-Medical School." During much of the year house-staff members work along with medical students and professors. Patterns of responsibility in University Hospital weave the intern and his role partners into the fabric of the joint medical school-hospital in ways that imply a continuation of medical school influence and provide occasions for house-staff members to identify with medical education. Some have opportunities to act in the teacher's role and learn that the role becomes them.

Thirty-seven other specialty interns and more than 157 specialty residents also reported for training on this first of July.[1] Eighteen interns were taking the straight medical internship; the rest were in straight surgical, pediatrics, or pathology internships. Many of these interns would stay for extended training through a number of years. Some of the interns had been in the hospital as students in the affiliated medical school, a fact in this environment that contributes consistency of influence toward extended training and specialization.

After much correspondence with the hospital, the intern and his wife had rented a small apartment in an old building that stood within three blocks of the hospital. This was one of the hospital-owned apartment buildings in the neighborhood where apartments were rented to house-staff members for between $50 and $95 a month. The intern's beginning salary was $143 a month with partial maintenance. By 1968 the salary was $375 with partial maintenance.[2] He would pay for his meals and room in the hospital.

Reporting early in the morning, the intern received a mimeographed schedule of house-staff assignments for the entire year. Four of his assignments were on private and semiprivate services, where attending physicians would be principally responsible for their own cases but where the intern would do the initial examination and history. Prepared by the chief res-

ident on medicine, the schedule showed nine forty-day assignments, and located him and another intern on one of the
medical ward services—beginning now.

The assistant resident assigned to the intern's ward had
worked as a medical student, an intern, a resident, and a research fellow at University Hospital, and was taking another
year as an assistant resident to "brush up" before going into
practice. He greeted the intern warmly. "Welcome to A-I.
Where are you from? That's a fine place. Is Dr. X. still there?
They've turned out some excellent research."

Values of the hospital, as well as the type of medical practice
it represents, were communicated many times during the first
day of internship. Early in the day the intern went to a separate
ward within the medical service where he would work closely
with another medical intern and an assistant resident. In his
greeting, the resident had established the academic orientation
of the hospital and all the other teaching centers that produced
research results. At the same time, the resident acknowledged
his acceptance of the intern as "one of us," someone from
another "good place." Through the year the close ties between
several medical schools and their renowned hospitals throughout
the country will be reinforced many times. Some of the attending physicians will know more about what another full-time
man in their specialty is doing in a distant city than they know
about what is happening in another specialty in their own hospital.

After introducing the intern to the head nurse who was in
the nursing station with them, the assistant resident asked if
the intern had seen much of the rest of the hospital. The intern
said, "No, and I don't know if I could find my way back from
the place we met this morning. What about this schedule they
gave me?"

The assistant resident went over the floor assignments, explaining which ones were private and which were wards. He
explained that there were two interns and one resident on most
floors. Interns would alternate twenty-four-hour duty, admitting
all patients when they were "on." Patients they admitted would
be theirs. The assistant resident continued, "I do a second

work-up on the patients you have admitted. The first work-up has to be the full one. The second may be a little bit briefer . . . My responsibility will be to check charts and see things are pretty much in order."

Before time for a coffee break, the intern already had been introduced to themes that will run through this day and later —that medical work in this hospital is subject to detailed review, and that careful medical histories and physical examinations are expected and that this is one of a company of very special research and teaching centers in the country.

For well over half of the intern's year, he will work with the ward patients for whom he will carry primary responsibility. For all of these patients, and some private ones on one special service, a resident will replicate the intern's admission work— take a history, examine and enter his findings after those of the intern in the patient's chart. And for a few months, a medical student will also write his findings in the chart of this same patient. The student's notes, while not an official part of the chart, will also be available for consideration.

The assistant resident continued, "As far as lab work goes, that will be your responsibility for all your patients. The guy who admits does admitting lab work (simple and routine work such as blood counts, guiacs, etc.). We may have to help each other when things get rushed for any one of us. Later in the year we will have students and they will help a lot with this work. But in one way we can move faster without them because we won't have to stop to do any teaching . . . Miss A. will show us around."

The resident introduced Miss A., the head nurse, with some pleasant asides. Typical of a large portion of graduate nurses at University Hospital, Miss A. was young, personable, and trained in the degree program affiliated with University Hospital. She described the functions and procedures of the drug, linen, and oxygen rooms as she showed the men from room to room. She said the floor clerk was "very good about calling for X-rays and taking care of things like that. You can depend on her to see that patients get up to X-ray as ordered." Then the nurse went over some forms, ending, "We have a form you have to sign for just about everything. But many of them you won't have to worry about, because we can fill them out for you, and all you have to do is sign them." Once again, solidarity is implied and the possible gains from staying in the good graces of a team member are suggested. At the same time the jocular comment about bureaucratic demands for forms expresses the attitudes of the medical team about expectations for priorities when needs of the bureaucracy run counter to goals of advancing knowledge.

The second intern who was to work on the same floor had arrived before the nurse started on the tour of the floor, so the assistant resident and the two interns started rounds together, as they would each morning. The assistant resident pulled the rolling chart rack toward the first room in which patients were to be seen. He took out a patient's chart, went through it, indicating the original history and physical findings, the shorter follow-up notes, nurses' notes, laboratory report entries, progress notes, and notes of consultants, adding, "Dr. Y. (chief of service) comes in and may write a note, or a consultant like someone from the eye group might enter a note . . . I will be around tonight and next week. But if anything of importance comes up and I am not on, call me *any* time." Another theme is introduced. Through the year the intern will hear many expressions in support of consultation and of candid admission of his own uncertainty. He will also find himself in situations where failure to ask for consultation carries unfortunate consequences and social disapproval of his colleagues.

After they had discussed all patients to be seen in a room, the three entered. When they approached the bedside of each patient, the assistant resident introduced the interns and they chatted briefly before the resident began the examination. In some cases, one or both of the interns listened to a chest sound, felt an abdomen, examined a foot, asked a few questions. On this first day the assistant resident initiated most of the action. However, each of the interns at some point suggested an added diagnostic procedure for some patient. Every time the assistant resident seemed very much interested and responded with, "Very good point," or "Good idea, we'll do it." He occasionally mentioned a research report related to a problem they discussed. Citation of the latest research findings and reports from diagnostic tests are acts frequently rewarded with admiration from house-staff members and sometimes also by a professor.

Patient census of the floor was not unusual—twenty-seven, male and female. Eventually, each intern would carry about fifteen staff patients on this assignment, and would admit an average of three patients a day when he was "on duty."

Two very sick patients were in private rooms, as was one disturbed, senile patient. The rest were in four-bed rooms. Rounds took almost two hours. The assistant resident said he thought they could finish rounds more quickly as they got their "own" patients (patients for whom they had performed the initial physical examination and history). The assistant resident added that he thought they should "make it a habit" to start rounds each morning "no later than 8:30 . . . bloods should be drawn before then."

The intern would discover that if he arrived late in the morning his group would also be late because they had waited for him. Time to start, time to finish rounds, time off for the coffee-break would be determined by *group* pace for the particular ward.

When the two interns and their assistant resident were about halfway through rounds, they stopped to have coffee in the ward's supply room. The room was crowded; a large coffee pot steamed cheerily, and one of the nurses had brought coffee cake. The assistant resident introduced the out-of-town intern. The other one seemed to know everyone, for he had served as a clinical clerk in the hospital; he was welcomed back as an intern. Talk between interns and residents was animated and highlighted by enthusiastic accounts of unusual findings, as when the hematology resident described results of a punch biopsy he had performed the previous week on a patient currently on this ward.* The hematologist said he knew of only one similar case reported in the literature.

---

* A punch biopsy is a method in which a small cylindroid piece of tissue for biopsy is removed by means of a special instrument that may be pierced directly into an organ, or through the skin or a small incision in the skin.

The chief resident for medicine dropped in, asking how the patient, Mrs. Z., was this morning. He discussed her briefly with the assistant resident, then told the interns, "You are starting in a good place; it is where I started." Then, as the group stood leaning against the narrow room's cupboards and sinks, he described a few of his experiences and his feelings of uncertainty during his first hectic week of internship.

The coffee-break lasted less than twenty minutes. Returning to their rounds, the assistant resident mentioned two of the patients who were "very interesting." One, a "medical museum," had been in and out of University Hospital over a number of years, and could almost "be depended on" to react in an unexpected way to medication. The assistant resident suggested, "Sometime when you have time, you should go through some of his charts. They are filled with useful information."

Throughout the year, the intern would identify several such patients and he would find that in conferences many, if not most, of the medical house-staff also had treated them or given them tests, during one of the patient's many admissions. These patients would be discussed informally before and after conferences, over coffee or lunch. Many were referred to and addressed by their first names, and they were among the patients that interns and residents in this environment called "interesting." In this setting, the patient with an unusual medical problem provides the intern a chance to gain special notice, and also special chances for learning something new. The second intern leafed through the patient's current chart and told of seeing this patient on a previous admission. He then described a case with some similar problems he had seen at University Hospital last year when he was doing his clinical work as a fourth-year student.

Later in the week, the intern would note that many doctors looked through patients' charts—consultants from other services, the chief resident, the chief of service, assistant residents, medical students and their professors. The visibility of chart entries tends to encourage interns in this setting to attend rather promptly to careful examination and history-taking for their charts. No one told the intern he should take time in the afternoon and evening to "study" charts, but within the first month of his internship he had heard of a fellow intern's embarrassment over ordering medication that would have caused an unfortunate reaction in the particular patient. The resident on the floor had caught the error before medication was given, and had suggested to the intern that he check through the chart more carefully so he would be alert to potential unusual reactions.

Rounds this first day were completed at about 11:30. Interns went back to the patients' rooms. The assistant resident went to the nursing station, recorded a finding on one of his patient's charts, then worked in the laboratory briefly. There was a hum of activity around the nursing area most of the day. It was the floor communication center, the place where records and messages were kept. Occasionally, a group of people in white coats appeared in the nursing station together, looked through a chart, discussed it for a few minutes, and then went to see a patient. These were various specialty groups who had been called in to consult on a case.

At about 12:15 the intern came into the nursing station, sat down with a deep sigh and said, "I don't even know where the drinking fountain is and I'm parched." The assistant resident hurried into the station, suggested the intern "might want to draw blood on Mr. B. and Miss C." The intern jumped up to follow the suggestion but reappeared almost immediately to look for a pipette and to check the patients' room numbers.

The assistant resident had been extremely busy all morning. He had arrived at 8:00 to make rounds and get acquainted with the patients, and he had been on the phone many times, either asking this ward's former assistant resident about a patient, or answering questions from the man who had taken over the assignment he had just left. Through the year, residents would move to a different unit every forty-five days, so that after this rushed first of July either the interns or the resident on each assignment would already be familiar with all cases on the floor. Even so, with each shift the intern would experience certain anxiety as he faced new patients, nurses he had not worked with before, an intern he may or may not have served with, and perhaps a resident with whom he had not worked.

Shortly after 12:30, the intern asked the assistant resident if he could go home for lunch and, "When I go home, I would sign out to you?" The assistant resident answered, "Just tell someone on the floor where you are going so they know where to reach you." When the intern returned, some forty minutes later, he exclaimed to an observer that his furniture had arrived "from home, and they dumped it on the sidewalk." He seemed bewildered—especially about the fact that the movers would not accept his check—and he added wistfully, "It seems pretty impersonal." A large city and a large hospital presents the intern with many impersonal exchanges but some of the impersonality he meets before his arrival and in the first days will later be balanced by the small groups that work together closely within each specialty.

All medical house-staff members gathered in the medical library at 1:15, the appointed time for their staff meeting. Doctors sat around the massive table in handsome black captain's chairs, each with the hospital insignia and the date "1771" inscribed on its back—a date many speakers mentioned during the day. Eventually, most members of the house staff would be presented with one of these chairs—after two years' service—a solid symbol of experience in one of the country's longest established hospitals.

The chief resident in medicine introduced each of the house-staff members, old and new, indicating where newcomers were from, and how the specialty residents would relate to the work of the interns. The chief resident mentioned that one of the new interns had had a previous internship in pathology. Two of the "first-year" assistant residents in medicine had previous residency rotations through this service at University Hospital, and were taking a second year of rotation to "brush up." A third on this same "first-year" resident rotation schedule had already been a resident in an out-of-state university hospital the year before.

The chief resident described the hospital's program, emphasizing the goal "to develop a free exchange of ideas." Then he discussed "teaching responsibilities" and "research obligations" as well as patient service. He urged the interns to feel free to ask for help or advice "even if you just want us to hold your hand . . . You would not be here if we did not think you could get through it all fine." He announced rounds and conferences held regularly on the service—chief of service's "grand rounds" Thursday morning, chief resident's rounds Tuesday and Friday afternoons, chief of service's work rounds Wednesday morning, attendings' rounds twice a week. Then there were the special conferences—neurology, hematology, dermatology, radiology, and cardio-vascular conference, gastrointestinal conference, and the clinical pathological conference. He reminded the group that their own daily work rounds on ward services would "begin not later than 8:30. That means the interns have to have all bloods drawn before then. Attendings or consultants are not to interrupt these rounds. Let me know if they do."

The out-of-town intern would later take for granted the primacy of scheduled teaching rounds that were not to be interrupted. He was at first surprised when a doctor with a private practice appeared during rounds to talk about one of his cases, and the assistant resident suggested the senior physician wait until after rounds were finished.

This acknowledgment of priority of house-staff teaching over attending physician's convenience in University Hospital makes explicit some recognition of the importance and prestige of the house-staff group vis-à-vis the attending physician who is in private practice. Implications of such primacy of house-staff's daily rounds come into relief as we hear other comments about attending physicians. The chief resident, speaking of attending physicians, commented, "You should keep them informed, for they are here to help and they are also here to learn. Let's not set out to trap them."

This seeming recognition that house staff is likely to see the attending physicians as almost "fair game" and "in season" when they appear on University Hospital wards to teach, suggests how widespread may be the inclination in this environment to devalue a senior physician who seems peripheral to the medical-school learning environment, and a few or many years away from full-time learning of the latest medical-scientific advances.

After the chief resident spoke, he left the room to usher in the chief of service whom he had referred to with deference as "The Professor." Distinguished, grey-haired though not yet forty, and immaculate in his white coat, the chief stood as he spoke to his new staff members. He mentioned the long, illustrious history of the hospital, emphasized advantages, privileges, and responsibilities of the intern at University Hospital. He warned against a house-staff member ever taking any outside work during his appointment in this hospital. Later as the intern told a friend about his work at University Hospital, he said he didn't think anyone could possibly have time to violate this regulation. Scheduled rounds, conferences, plus his work with patients, kept him too busy to take on anything else. In many other hospitals it is not unusual for house-staff members to supplement their income with outside work.

The senior physician repeated his chief resident's assurance that senior and junior members of the staff were always there to help when needed. "You will soon find that there is not anyone around here who does not need to know something. You already know more about some things than some of the staff, and soon you will know more. Preserve a very precious system— graduated specialization . . . call the assistant resident, the resident, and only then the attending." The chief of service also reported "Over two hundred significant published reports from here last year . . . over one million dollars spent on research." Teaching and research were frequently and effectively presented as primary values by several speakers this first day of internship. Comprehensive patient care is also assumed to be a priority concern in this hospital, but this value did not receive as much reinforcement as did research and teaching.

Returning to the ward, the intern discovered there was a new patient on the floor and one more yet to be admitted. He was "on" today, and so was responsible for work-up on all admissions and for calls during the night. The assistant resident had said he would probably average "two or three admissions a day" on a ward such as this, but fewer for a while until the assistant resident and his interns "had time to clear out the ward and make way for new ones." The assistant resident explained that the medical resident assigned to emergency room duty for two weeks admits *all* ward patients to the medical floors, and "he can't admit if we don't have vacant beds."

The out-of-town intern had been a clinical clerk in a metropolitan university hospital where patient admissions were not screened for teaching purposes. He expressed surprise when a resident, serving as admitting officer in the hospital emergency room, came on the floor and apologized to his fellow house-staff members for having admitted one case he was afraid was "not too interesting." But later in the year the intern would find himself expressing his own annoyance to an admitting officer for having sent up an "uninteresting case."[3]

At 3:30 the intern rushed off to the next meeting on his schedule—this one a joint session for new house-staff members from all departments—held in a large surgical amphitheater. A doctor, "associate director for professional services," chaired the meeting as house staff leaned forward to listen from their straight, high-backed wooden "pews." The secretary-treasurer spoke first, informing interns, not for the first time, that they were "joining a proud company." Another pervasive theme of the initiation days is the recognition of University Hospital's proud history, long tradition, and its prestige within the network of medical schools and hospitals. We shall see that this recognition provides a solid base and enough security to support the kinds of innovative effort demanded for scientific advance.

The tradition is glorified in speeches, symbolized by the ubiquitous founding date of the hospital. A way of life is transmitted from one year's house officers to the next. Continuity is thus assured by extended training and by teamwork and by emphasis on solidarity in the proud company of University Hospital physicians.

The director of nurses, chief pharmacist, and record librarian each gave a prepared speech, locating their departments in the hospital structure, citing significant regulations concerning their work, and offering to help the interns. Among the speakers, only the record librarian, the secretary-treasurer, and the associate director's assistant did not appear in long white coats, as though the coat were a symbol of some separating line between medical and lay staff at University Hospital.

For the fourth time in the day, the intern was invited to ask for help when it was needed. The associate director said, "Sometimes in anxiety to do a job and to convince your superiors you know what you are doing, (you) can get into trouble if (you) do not ask for help. We would urge you . . . if you find yourself in a situation where you feel you are unable to cope . . . please ask the people next to you for help. As a matter of fact, they will think more of you because you have exercised good judgment in calling for help." In this environment asking for help confirms the status system. It allows the intern's seniors to do what they are supposed to do—to teach. The intern in a sense can also show that he "knows his place" and that he "belongs" because he wants to learn.

Through the year, the intern would come upon many occasions when house-staff members and professors alike would admit their own uncertainty and the limits to their knowledge, and many occasions when such acknowledgment would be affirmed. This explicit advice to seek assistance would receive much confirming support from action as well as words.

At 4:30, after a few brief announcements covering pay dates and the location of the mail room, each house-staff member filed down the steep aisles of the amphitheater, passed a table to receive his large packet of information—a forty-four-page manual of information for house officers, two booklets on City Department of Health regulations, a booklet on malpractice suits, an illustrated brochure on the history of the hospital, a cloth-bound formulary, and six pages of sample forms for the intern's use.

At 4:45 P.M., the intern had finished his first day as it had been scheduled for him and his fellow interns. As he came down the elevator to return to his assigned floor, he looked at the large packet of reading material and said, "Will I ever have time to read it? I have two new patients to admit tonight, and there are so *many* interesting patients on the ward!" This intern would find that the assistant resident on his floor stayed on late that night with him. Before the assistant resident left at midnight, they had called in the cardiologist resident, and the three of them worked together over a critically ill patient. The young man who had arrived at University Hospital early that morning had become a member of the house staff.

Values and Their Reinforcements

Both at University Hospital and at Community Hospital, senior physicians and other hospital spokesmen at orientation meetings offer interns clues about the norms and values of their hospital, and at the same time provide some measure of consistency between the ideal and the reality interns will face in their particular hospital. Each hospital offers its interns somewhat different possibilities for the future. Each encourages different patterns of interaction and communication, variations in sources of rewards and punishments, and objective situations the intern will most often meet. Such situations are the stuff out of which value climates are created; and the values of that creation in turn become a part of the social reality that influences action as well as attitudes.

Values, while often generated out of real interests as well as by objective situations, take on a reality and force of their own.[4] They become the orienting principles, the rationale behind action, the life perspectives, the sentiments, the themes, the spirit that gives coherence to behavior.[5] The first impulse to social action may be given by interests as practical and real as money, power, convenience, personal or social comfort. But ideals, values, and principles lend wings to these real interests by justifying and giving spiritual meaning to them.[6] "[Mankind] wants to have a good conscience as he pursues his life-interests. And in pursuing them he develops his capacities to the highest extent only if he believes that he serves a higher rather than a purely egoistic purpose. Interests without such "spiritual wings" are lame; but on the other hand, ideas can win out in history only if and insofar as they are associated with real interest."[7]

Much of the behavior of physicians is inexplicable without the concept of values. The beliefs that human life is precious, that it is better to search and improve than to accept what is, that scientific investigation is good, and that human suffering should be alleviated are matters of faith, and not subject to test and proof.[8] Physicians rise in the middle of the night, pour over research reports, forego a weekend off, attend conferences, buy books, not only to gain more money and prestige but also in response to ethical premises. The consequences of beliefs and values are real and measurable. Lives are saved; people are relieved of pain. Scientific advances are made and health is improved.

Values are general, and their lack of precision provides necessary leeway. One can hold to commitments and sustain belief and consensus in spite of contradictory demands and in spite of occasional contradictory behavior that goes unsanctioned.[9]

The general value orientations that support the physician's work are upheld alike in University Hospital and Community Hospital, and they are upheld in both places by work and action as well as by declaration. Within these broad and general commitments of medicine to saving life, searching for ways to prolong life, relieving suffering, and restoring health, there are variations in minor value themes between the two hospitals. Thus, at University Hospital, such values as "tradition," "graduated specialization," "advancing knowledge," are presented to the intern as important values in his hospital starting with his first orientation meetings. "Friendly atmosphere," and "individual initiative" provide the minor value themes at Community Hospital, beginning with the orientation dinner. It is these variations of value themes that we will attend to. Though on the surface they may seem extraneous to the "real interests" and the "bigger" values, they may imply differences of some consequence for the developing physician.

On graduation day at the University Hospital medical school, interns and residents gather at hospital windows to watch parts of the outdoor graduation ceremonies, some of them recalling the day when they were graduated on the same grounds.[10] The hospital adds its own ceremonies to keep alive the vital memories of medical school, and repeated references to the early founding of the hospital help to emphasize its "proud history."

"Grand rounds" in the teaching center are formal and dignified. In addition to a rich, cognitive content, they offer an impressive ritual of professional behavior. At one grand rounds in medicine, interns presented cases in detail from a podium, and each presentation was followed by invited, formal discussants. Just before the first patient was brought in by a nurse, a roomful of physicians and nurses snuffed out their cigarettes, as if on signal from a cloister bell. A white-coated professor set the tone of the meeting, affirming the image of the physician's respect for his patient, as he first put the patient at ease, and only then discussed the case. Discussion from the floor was held for most part by professors, some of whom reported first-hand experience with related research. In such conferences at major teaching centers medical standards are established and supported somewhat as the military academies largely set the standards of behavior for the whole military profession.[11] Major conferences at university hospitals brings to mind Durkheim's phrase, "Just as the priest is the interpreter of his god, the teacher is the interpreter of the great moral ideas of his time and of his country."[12] Grand rounds at University Hospital suggest that the physician-teacher serves as an interpreter of the moral ideas of his profession.

These grand rounds continue the "sustaining value-environment provided by the medical school" as Merton describes it. "The great tradition in medicine is in large part a tradition of commitment to the search for improved, and therefore changing, ways of coping with the problems of the sick. It is in this sense that respect for medical tradition is an enduring part of the culture of medical education. Frequent ceremonies serve to keep alive a sense of the core-values of medicine as these are exemplified in the achievements of those who have gone before."[13]

One medical educator spelled out faculty awareness of the function of ritual in medical school: "The Faculty Council decided again to dress in the traditional university cap and gown. To some, these costumes may seem old-fashioned or unattractive, but to most of us, they symbolize a fact of the highest importance, that you and we are part of a great tradition of Western culture—of the university as the seat of inquiry, as the center of new ideas, as the caretaker of the great ideas of the past, as the center of honest teaching and of scientific research."[14] Some rituals at University Hospital provide "symbolic acts of solidarity" that draw physicians together in belief that they are a "proud company."[15] Such experiences support a conviction of the rightness of science and its methods. The backdrop of prestige and tradition at University Hospital may also provide a stable setting and some needed security for consistent and pervasive emphasis on innovation through science, and on never ending replacement of the old by the new in scientific progress.[16] Charles Cooley estimated the importance of orthodoxy for innovation: "Thus all innovation is based on conformity, all heterodoxy on orthodoxy, all individuality on solidarity. Without the orthodox tradition in biology, for instance, under the guidance of which a store of ordered knowledge had been collected, the heterodoxy of Darwin, based on a reinterpretation of this knowledge, would have been impossible. And so in art, the institution supplies a basis to the very individual who rebels against it."[17]

Tradition and ceremonies can provide needed reassurance for professionals: "the people who got it into their heads that anything formal is cold [do not realize] that ceremonial may be the cloak that warms the freezing heart, that a formula may be the firm stick upon which the trembing limbs may lean; that it may be a house in which one may decently hide himself until he has the strength and courage to face the world again."[18] Ritual tends to develop in occupations such as medicine where there are great and unavoidable risks.[19]

Internship at Community Hospital: A Friendly Place

In the late afternoon before the first of July, an intern from an out-of-state medical school reported to the administrative office of the 360-bed Community Hospital, the larger of the two hospitals in a suburban town. He, like his counterpart at University Hospital, had arrived at his hospital through the National Intern Matching Plan. But the Community Hospital man had selected a rotating internship.[20]

Community Hospital spreads out over a low hill, displaying examples of a number of years of architecture and changing attitudes in the community toward a hospital's accepted function. A few isolated frame buildings date from the late 1800's, the major group from 1910, with dark red brick and porticos and one recent glass-walled addition. The buildings stand among frame houses on a tree-lined street. Ramps connecting hospital buildings adhere to contours of the hill and in one place enclose a bit of land, carefully tended with flowers and trees.

As the eight connected buildings of Community Hospital spread out into their immediate neighborhood, so lines of interaction and potential influence interlock the local community and its hospital. Most attending physicians who teach interns and residents have their offices out in the community. Many nurses are married, work part time, and have significant obligations outside the hospital. Volunteers in the hospital cast other personal lines that tie the hospital into its local community.

The local press is eager for news of developments, additions, and advances in "its" hospital. The hospital's hospitality shop is a bright and cheerful place where families of patients, the hospital administrator, volunteers, lab technicians, nurses, interns, and chiefs of services all go for a coffee break, tea, or lunch. Friendly exchanges in the informal shop draw lay and medical people together. A phone on a window sill allows physicians to respond to a page or to call their answering services while they wait for their food.

During most of the year, two residents and ten rotating general interns share house-staff duties. One of the residents was scheduled to leave by September; two of the ten interns had not yet arrived. Four of the five medical students who work somewhat as interns during the summer had arrived; one was not due until August.

The Community Hospital intern was married; he and his wife had visited the hospital some weeks before, had seen their apartment, and had talked about plans for it with Mrs. M., the administrative secretary of the hospital. Mrs. M. assigns apartments, sees that they are freshly cleaned and furnished, even to a small supply of linens, "so (the newly arrived intern and his family) . . . could be comfortable the first few nights, whether or not any of their own things arrived." She will hand them their regular pay checks, take care of problems of apartment management, relay messages, even remind them to pick up their uniforms to save them time when they get absent-minded. She is pleasant, energetic, and has been at the hospital for over thirty years.

The friendly atmosphere of the hospital, the pleasant quality of the community, and the low-rent apartments are all included as extra selling points for Community Hospital as it competes for interns. The hospital and its administration do become involved in the life of the intern and his family. Some secondary characteristics of the intern take on special importance, corresponding to the intern's interest in secondary characteristics of the hospital. In this situation where more people know more about the life situation of patient and doctor and nurse, the house-staff's low rank, relative to many of the patients he sees, can become a problem. In the smaller community and friendly place, style of life becomes a relevant attribute of the intern today and also later, if he stays to practice in the community.

Possibly related to hospital competition for interns is the willingness of its administration to make individual arrangements for interns; to be flexible, for example, with the intern who needs to arrive later than the first of July to start his internship; or for the intern whose wife wants to work in the hospital; or for the intern who wants extra surgical experience after he completes his internship requirements.

Mrs. M. had a small packet of material for each intern, including a spiral-bound notebook that held a collection of information selected to help him settle into Community Hospital personally, as well as professionally. There was a map of the town—"compliments of the C. Savings Bank"—an attending-staff schedule with assignments and telephone numbers, a roster of nurses in the hospital, plus some outside numbers—ambulances, churches, florists, home telephone numbers of the director of nurses, the pathologists, pharmacist, and administrative secretary. There were also phone numbers of medical examiners, Alcoholics Anonymous, post office, railroad station, and state troopers, and some seventeen local undertakers and eleven convalescent homes. The intern at Community Hospital is presented with many reminders of the hospital's orientation to the community. He is also reminded of the financial rewards that can follow if he becomes accepted in the community.

A memorandum from the administrative secretary began, "We hope you will find your living quarters adequate and a pleasant base for a happy year." A notebook also held sample forms and separate sections of information from the chief of each of the four services, and one signed by the director of nurses. Mrs. M. gave the intern a house-staff roster and a rotation schedule for the month, covering a short time, as the hospital administrator said, "in order to allow for adjustments after the whole staff has arrived and settled in."

The house-staff roster showed medical schools from which each of the house-staff members was graduated: two of them came from one state university medical school; one was from a major school in the Midwest; one from a large metropolitan school; one from a smaller school in the South; and one from a Canadian medical school. One had come from a medical school in Amsterdam, one from Lausanne, one from Basel, one from Rome, one from Capetown, one from Manila. The five medical students who were serving a summer clerkship came from still different schools. All of the American or Canadian-trained interns were married. Two of the house-staff members were women—one an intern and one a medical student working for the summer.

The intern's new apartment was in a one-story building designed as the hospital's isolation unit before medicine had gained control over some infectious diseases. Now, to meet changing community needs, the building was sectioned into living units that opened onto a small courtyard where tricycles and bicycles were often parked. Another group of apartments nestled together in a recently converted, ample, old frame house. All apartments were rented to staff for $10 per room a month. In 1958 beginning salary of the intern was $100 with full maintenance. By 1968 beginning salary in this hospital was $433 with partial maintenance. The hospital administrator and the administrative trainee, and all house-staff members lived on the hospital grounds; their children played together. The chief anesthetist lived "a few houses down" on a nearby street.

At about 6:30 P.M. the intern, neatly dressed in a business suit, found his way to the staff cafeteria for the orientation dinner-meeting which had been called by the hospital administrator. A few of the newcomers (whom the intern soon learned were medical students doing summer work) and his fellow interns were gathering in the hallway. Standing near the entrance to the cafeteria, the hospital administrator introduced interns to each other and to the attending physicians as they began to arrive. The administrator was easy and pleasant, and he remembered where each intern had come from, and identified the people he introduced to each other, offering a starting point for exchange before moving to the next introduction.

Each person picked up his own dinner in the cafeteria line and seated himself at the tables arranged to form a large, hollow square. The food was attractively displayed and good. People seated themselves in pairs or trios, following introductions or conversations initiated in the cafeteria line or before. The two women physicians sat together, as did the two interns who came from the same medical school. As attending physicians arrived, they filled in spaces between small clusters of house-staff members. Paper place-mats on the tables carried the message, "Greetings from the many hands and many skills serving you at Community Hospital," and below the message a chart presented the personnel of the hospital in cartoon form, giving the number of people in each position, and placing the patient in the center of all activities.

The administrator started the meeting by introducing each of the approximately twenty-five people around the table. He hesitated at no name and identified all the senior people in some detail. "Miss M., administrative secretary, is in charge of paychecks . . . shoulder to cry on . . . in charge of housing . . . Dr. S., there, in the loud coat . . . director of the Educational Committee."

The administrator said he would talk for the rest of the evening, but he expected the interns to remember only the general ideas and *who* said different things. "But before I start talking, I want to ask Dr. Y. to talk to you. He is wanting to get away for a vacation so he will talk first and leave." The emphasis on the individual rather than on regulation and rules was one theme of the welcoming speeches.

The administrator, after introductions, asked each chief of service to speak. No one had an obviously prepared speech. No one mentioned the "proud history" of the hospital—a theme in some of the University Hospital orientation comments. Interns were urged to take advantage of potential learning experiences available to them. The attending physicians were identified as a present source of advice, help, information, and a future source of recommendations. One physician said, "We hope you are impressed with the fact that this is a general rotating internship, and that this means that you have the opportunity to gain some experience in different fields and decide what you want to specialize in. We do not feel, of course, that you will be proficient as surgeons, etc. But how proficient you become, how much experience you gain from each service will be *up to you.* Dr. G., here, had become interested in OB-GYN and he has gotten a good deal of experience in it."[21] The head of the pathology laboratory said, "We welcome you to come to the lab any time. We will depend for the most part on your coming to us." The administrator said, "The attending will respond to you in proportion to your interest. When you are in OB, if you are slovenly and lazy . . . you will get mighty few deliveries to do. Several years ago, an intern so impressed the attendings that he delivered eighty babies in eight weeks."

One of the chiefs of service, in his informal comments, emphasized his wish that interns feel free to ask questions in his department. Another physician stressed the importance of becoming a part of the hospital community. "I believe there are excellent opportunities here for you. I believe both professional and social contacts can help you develop as physicians . . . I hope you will try to become friends as well as pupils."

On July 1, the morning following the orientation dinner, the intern came into the hospital's auditorium shortly after nine. Most of the others were already gathered there and beginning to get acquainted. The hospital administrator arrived to hand out sticker-badges and to suggest that new members use them for identification: "They will stay on till July 4 and by that time most everybody will know you." The administrator left shortly, leaving in charge the resident who only yesterday had been an intern.

The resident conducted the interns through the hospital. When they arrived in the emergency room, they were introduced to the surgical resident who described work on emergency duty. The intern assigned there to day-duty for July separated himself from the group to stand behind the high "desk" of the nursing station; two interns talked quietly together; one moved away to peer into some of the emergency rooms. The resident continued his orientation remarks. "Don't be embarrassed or ashamed if you are doing something and they [nurses] tell you, 'Doctor, that is something that should not be done.' After a while, you will know our procedures and they [nurses] . . . will not have to tell you. You will usually be informed before the patient arrives. They [nurses] decide with you what should be done for the patient. For the first two months . . . [the nurse] sees that the surgical resident will be here with you, and on some cases they will call the attending physician."

The resident showed the new house-staff members the EKG room where a technician demonstrated use of the machines, employing one of the interns as a volunteer subject. As they moved to different departments, they chatted together, finding out more about their colleagues; two discovered they had friends in common. Occasionally, a hospital page on the loudspeaker system would call an intern to his assigned floor. At each stop, the resident introduced the interns to hospital personnel, commenting on how they would be able to help the house-staff members in their work.

Arriving at the front entrance of the hospital, near the record room, the resident used a large diagram on the hospital wall to describe the spatial location of buildings and departments. One intern asked what the building labeled "M. Hall" was. It was the nurses' quarters, and one of the group commented on the importance of getting oriented.

After they had gone to see their rooms in the hospital and picked up mail that was waiting for them, they went back to the record room. As the house-staff members stood in the record room looking at the patient charts and the dictating machines, an intern asked whether discharge summaries were dictated or written out in longhand. The resident said they were usually written out "because they . . . [are] *usually so short . . . there isn't need to dictate them.*" The resident answered other questions from interns and continued talking about charts. "You better do . . . [write-ups of examinations and history taken on admission] . . . quickly, because if you are behind over fifteen of them they withhold your pay check. You are better off to do them as fast as you can and not let them pile up."

Before the house-staff group left the record room, one intern asked where "old records are kept." The resident, apparently assumed the question referred to records waiting to be dictated by the interns. He said, "You check here; they are by the intern's name." Two interns exchanged glances and the second one rephrased the question, "But what about records on patients who are admitted here for a second time?" The resident said that they should be on the floor "or you can call for them." The intern will learn very quickly in this environment that patient charts are not the focus of learning and teaching or the vital communication instrument they had been in the affiliated hospital where he had his clinical experience as a fourth year student.

Just seven house-staff members were left on the "tour of the hospital" by the time it arrived at surgery. The surgical resident reappeared and described procedures there. He went through a "dress rehearsal" for surgery, explaining in detail the length of scrub-time required, and accepted practices for preparing to enter surgery. After the demonstration, he took the group to the floor's small lounge and showed them the refrigerator and its ample supply of soft drinks for physicians working on surgery. In the recovery room the surgical resident introduced the new house-staff members to the nurse in charge, and asked her a few questions about the number of patients who might be there on an average day. An attending physician came into the recovery room to see his patient and the surgical resident introduced the attending to the group, "Dr. Y. is an authority on urinary problems. He will speak to you on Wednesday about catheterization." The attending acknowledged the introduction in a friendly way and said he would see them soon. As the interns and the surgical resident left the recovery room, the nurse who had talked with them followed the interns into the hall, saying, "I hope you like it . . . it is kind of spread out and maybe a little confusing at first . . . you can always get a cup of coffee in that room in the corner."

By noon the last of the interns had gone their separate ways—some to their nearby apartments for lunch, some to their individual assignments. Just before 1:30, when the surgical orientation meeting was scheduled to begin, the two residents and only one third of the new interns had arrived. The atmosphere was relaxed, and both audience and the attending surgeon who was holding the meeting shared amusement as two latecomers burst into the room, looking flustered. The attending surgeon had asked the surgical resident to page all house-staff members, inviting them to the meeting. Some five or ten minutes later he asked for another page, adding, "and this time drop the word 'invited.'" The latecomers had appeared almost immediately and hurried to seat themselves.

The attending surgeon discussed some problems most frequently encountered in the emergency room—and he seemed to welcome questions from the house staff. He announced that a monthly journal meeting would he held in the homes of attending physicians. "I think this takes some of the onus off evening meetings . . . Having gone through an internship which was rather rugged, I know how you can miss time to read and keep up; this plan may help you." It is not unusual to hear attending physicians suggest that they worked harder when they were interns and residents than present interns do. But such comments seem more frequent in community hospitals that do have to be careful about demanding so much work from interns that one year's group interns would discourage others from following them.

The surgeon read some notes from the nursing staff, making known their regulations for emergency room duty. Several times during the orientation day, the incoming interns were directed to attend to information from nurses.

The surgical meeting, the last for the day, was finished by 2:30, and the intern went into the hospital's coffee shop to relax for a moment before going to the floors to which he was assigned. He explained to the observer that he didn't have any ward patients yet, but that he did have about thirty private patients. He added that he would have to "read all their charts and be familiar with all of them . . . [and] make rounds and see them." His evident surprise, when the observer asked whether he thought he would see these private cases "except in emergency" suggested the zeal of a new recruit. No one of the speakers in any of the meetings had suggested the intern would be responsible for this kind of follow-up with private patients. House-staff members interviewed later in their year described obligations to private patients as limited to admission work-up and any emergencies that arose while the intern was "on duty." Later, at the orientation meeting that nurses hold for the interns, a nursing supervisor described the intern's responsibility as limited to initial admission work (physical and histories) except in emergencies. Six days after this intern's statement of what he "would have to do," he told an observer that he had not yet "had time" to go on rounds with any attending physicians when they came in to see their private patients, and he added, "I have not had time to make rounds myself."

The intern was not "on duty" this first night so he went home for the evening at about 6 o'clock, having finished three of the seven admission work-ups waiting to be completed for private patients. Within his first three nights as an intern, he had served on duty one night when a nurse called him to see a patient who had gone into cardiac arrest. The intern learned from working with the night supervisor of nurses just how much assistance an experienced and knowledgeable nurse could give—and how much an attending physician could seem to trust her. Without appearing to assume authority, the supervisor asked the intern if he wanted her to arrange for oxygen, and "agreed" that he should call the patient's physician. She also mentioned something the physician usually wanted done in such cases. Except for these "suggestions" she stood by him and followed orders with dispatch. Later, when the senior physician arrived he com-

plimented the intern on his handling of the case. At the nurses'
orientation meeting for house staff, held later in the week, the
night supervisor used this intern's experience as a "good example" of work with private patients. "Dr. D. did just the right
thing. He instituted emergency measures and got in touch with
the attending."

Differences in Orientation and Values

The setting of "grand rounds" exemplifies the difference between Community Hospital and University Hospital in value
climates. At University Hospital the traditional steeply banked
medical auditorium was filled with professionals, mostly in
white coats and uniforms. At Community Hospital, a large
room with folding chairs held physicians, some in sport jackets,
some in uniform and a few in green surgical gowns.

Community Hospital grand rounds through the year were less
formal than those in the larger hospital. For example, one day
a house-staff member stood at ease near the front of the room
to present a case, and presentation was briefer than any observed
at grand rounds in University Hospital. For discussion of one
case an attending physician, dressed for surgery, stood at his seat
to give a brief history, then went out into the hall himself to
bring in the patient whose case he had presented.

The nature of the work schedules of attending physicians at
Community Hospital heightens awareness that time is a precious
commodity. The number of formal rounds and the contemplative discussions of multiple possibilities and probabilities are
reduced. The comparative brevity of case presentation may also
reflect differences in the kind of case often presented in an environment where patient admissions are not screened for teaching purposes, and where there are fewer highly specialized teams
to become involved with a case. This helps the hospital to handle diagnostic work-ups with dispatch—something that busy
patients may desire. But at the same time, this brevity has implications for what interns come to consider the "right" amount
of information for discussion—or for action.

There was more free-flowing discussion and questioning by
local physicians who were attendings, but less citation of "la-

test findings," and less protocol than at University Hospital. Also, discussions in the smaller hospital concentrated relatively more on immediate problem-solving (medical and administrative), and on what "usually happens with these cases," concretely, rather than on what might happen in the abstract.

The ethos of friendliness and informality appears to arise in part from requirements for flexibility and individual arrangements. In a hospital where most senior physicians have their offices out in the community, there is more obvious need to rely on the good will of nurses, interns, and other workers to care for patients and to call the attending in an emergency, but not to make a nuisance of calling. With little external power for control one may be made aware of the advantage to be gained from sympathetic understanding of people in the hospital.

Attending physicians at Community Hospital must establish relations with hospital staff members who are willing to help out—at times beyond formal demands of a given hospital position. In a similar way, the individual intern at Community Hospital may become aware that he needs to attract favorable attention of individual attending physicians and the *volunteered* help of nurses, if he is to gain maximum benefits from his training.

When Community Hospital house-staff members were asked to rank attributes they used when judging fellow house-staff members, three fourths attached "great importance" to "ability to work" effectively with nurses and technicians. Every house-staff member indicated such interpersonal ability was at least of some importance. University Hospital house-staff members more often relegated this ability to "minor importance." These differences are consistent with the apparently greater significance of nurses and other nonphysicians in the experience of the Community Hospital intern compared with its significance for the University Hospital intern. The differences are also consistent with the smaller hospital's emphasis on everybody getting along together.

One chief resident at University Hospital seemed to recognize the possibility that his orientation to evaluating attending physicians might differ from that used by some other physicians in other hospitals: "By 'good doctors' I *don't* mean the ones who have pleasant personalities, but the doctors who are well-trained." As this physician seemed to observe, "pleasantness," and kindness may not serve all medical goals well. The "nice person" and permissive atmosphere can interfere with excellence of performance and adherence to standards. The "kind" physician may, as University Hospital house-staff members suggested, "get too soft" and not order painful procedures. Commitment to the "friendly climate," and the "pleasant manner" may offer a rationale for diffuse relationships which in turn can make for special discomfort about enforcing demands.[22]

University Hospital offered many reminders of its close affiliation with its medical school—the presence of students, professors, research teams, portraits of educators from years gone by. Community Hospital alerted interns to ties with the local community—a map of the town, greetings from a savings bank, many volunteers, a coffee shop shared with patients, nurses, aides, chiefs of service, and administrators.

The University Hospital intern heard about the proud history and traditions, and an honored system of specialization to be preserved. The Community Hospital intern was directed toward personal initiative and moves he may make to get ahead on his own, and he heard much about the friendly atmosphere of his hospital.

The type of help available is different in the two hospitals. Asking for help in the University Hospital setting confirms the status system and identifies the intern as a doctor who "belongs" in a teaching center. At Community Hospital the intern is encouraged to see that senior physicians in his hospital can help him by allowing him valuable experience now and in the future by referring patients in the system of private practice around the hospital.

The University Hospital house staff is less transient than the one at Community Hospital. This provides continuity and development of closely knit specialty groups in the larger hospital. The relatively small staff at Community Hospital consists of a collection of physicians who are not expected to be together through many years of training. It is a small contingent with diverse backgrounds and individual professional needs. Sometimes these needs and the social support for initiative will impel the ambitious intern toward competitive, rather than cooperative activity with his peers.

University Hospital's older tradition, glorified by speech and symbol is to be made a "way of life," transmitted from year to year, day to day through continuity of staff. There are always several ranks of youthful "veterans" to confirm professional values and validate them through action.

Even the people who leave the house staff of University Hospital are likely to move to another similar hospital. Circulation of personnel between major teaching hospitals extends the medical academy and encourages development of a cosmopolitan elite—physicians who are in close touch with other physicians in their own specialty, in other university hospitals.

From the first of July onward, people and circumstances in Community Hospital direct the intern's attention to his own hospital, its local community, and to the individuals, both lay and medical, who can have relevance for his career, particularly, if he goes into practice in the community. Senior physicians at University Hospital cite the research contributions to the national medical community. Seniors at Community Hospital emphasize their hospital's contributions to the health care of the local community, and devote considerable attention to work in the emergency room.

The University Hospital intern spent most of his first day in the presence of other house-staff members and he moved mainly within his specialty's area in the hospital. The Community Hospital intern spent more of his first day as a solo physician—seeing patients, moving from one part of the hospital to the other.

The University Hospital intern learned to emphasize the team; the Community Hospital intern was taught to emphasize individual initiative. The University Hospital intern heard about research work and specialized areas of competency of his peers; the Community Hospital intern learned about individual characteristics and idiosyncrasies of some of the people with whom he would be working. He also began to hear about the personal and nonmedical aspects of nearly all people he met.

On the first day at University Hospital a resident complained to a fellow house-staff member that a ward patient who wasn't "interesting" had been admitted to his floor. And the intern learned that for the larger half of the year he would be working with the residents' selected patients who can offer interesting teaching material. The Community Hospital intern started the first day to do admission histories and physicals for private patients. He would continue through the year to see both private and ward patients as they arrived.

At University Hospital, the intern seemed bewildered by the impersonality of his transactions over furniture moving. At the Community Hospital, the intern was provided with linen "in case his furniture didn't arrive."

Senior physicians advised the University Hospital intern to call his resident first, then the chief resident, and to "preserve a precious system, graduated specialization." Senior physicians at Community Hospital told the intern how much trained and knowledgeable nurses might help him, and asked him *not* to hesitate about calling an attending directly.

The University Hospital intern was asked not to try to "trap the attendings" and was told that attendings were not to interrupt house-staff rounds. The Community Hospital intern was invited to "try to become friends as well as pupils with attendings" and he was reminded how much attendings might be able to help him toward experience now, and later, toward appointments or practice.

Charts were introduced to the intern in the large teaching hospital as a key focus in discussion about patients, and a source of valuable learning. Also, the intern there learned that his history and physical for newly admitted ward patients would be followed by the resident's history and physical, and at times by one of a medical student. At Community Hospital, the intern heard charts discussed as a part of his duties that *administration* might be interested in. He also heard "old records" referred to as admission work-ups an intern had yet to do, rather than (as at University Hospital) charts from a patient's previous admission.

As each of these two interns moved through the year toward

the following July first when he would be beginning his residency training, the directions that were implied this first day in each hospital would be repeatedly confirmed. The pressures and possibilities each hospital would offer its interns daily, and the hospital's hopes for its interns provide some of the material for them to create their own different constructions of a way of life in medicine.[23]

III | Traveling Different Paths

With each step toward professional position, processes of self-selection and social selection become increasingly apparent and significant for experience.[1] At each decision point, both the student and the educational institution selects, so that differences between people on the same training path narrow, and the distance between paths widens. The fervent stands made on each side of the two worlds in medicine, town and gown, illustrate one end-product of progressive divergence that takes place through career choice, selective recruitment in college, medical school, hospital, and the subsequent experiences in these institutions and the practice they foster.

Electing to take the longer road in medicine toward full specialized status, plus the fact of being thought suitable along the way, has a cumulative effect on attitudes. At each point the aspiring doctor has made "side bets" on behalf of the direction he has taken in training. If he elects the University Hospital specialty, training, and research route, he temporarily settles for less income, often less time off, and less comfortable living arrangements for himself and his family. He wagers that postponement will be worth it. Each decision along the way is a consequence of commitment, personality, and previous experience. But following that, the process of decision-making in areas where consequences are important, but not certain, generates urgency in the man's need to believe that his choice was right.[2]

On the other side, the physician who has gone the Community Hospital direction has some sense that he has taken less prestigeful training either because he was not admitted to a teaching center or because he decided to settle for more comfortable location, or for his hope to practice in that community. Whether that decision is dictated by his past record and earlier choices and chances, or whether it is a conscious decision at the end of medical school, such a physician may need to reassure himself that the way he has taken is right for him. The hospital where the physician has trained is a matter of import, for it can effect his subsequent chances for gaining affiliation in some hospitals.[3] In turn, the physician's career is partly conditioned by his hospital affiliation.

A tendency to proselytize often follows upon a final decision that was difficult to make. Having weighed bonuses and costs of different courses of action, the decision-maker is motivated to reassure himself that his was the right, perhaps the "only" valid decision.[4] Thus, physicians who have made successive career choices are liable to feel that their direction was not only best for them, but best for all in medicine. Attending physicians in each of these types of hospitals are often eloquent spokesmen for the direction of their own hospital as a promise for the future of medicine.

House-staff members of the two hospitals also made invidious comparisons that favored the orientation of their own hospital against "the other" kind of hospital and training. At University Hospital, physicians were quick to point out any inadequacies in records of diagnostic work that accompanied patients who had been referred to them from nearby community hospitals. At Community Hospital, interns and residents often claimed that men who trained in the large, renowned teaching hospitals were less effective in an emergency, or were cold and unaware of the person who was a patient. It is not that men in either hospital were blind to shortcomings in their own programs. In each hospital, some people were striving for improvement and were often candid in pointing out problems of their programs. But self-criticism in each hospital tended to end with a summary that reinforced the ultimate superiority of their hospital's training direction and orientations.

Compatibility Between Person and Environment

The type of students attracted to a hospital for their house-staff training is a vital element in the nature of the experiences the recruit will have there. In our nationwide survey of hospitals some 80 percent of the top students from the top American schools were in affiliated hospitals. Such students tend to be more oriented to careers in teaching and research.

Medicine is not alone in professions that develop separate career orientations through progressive selection and recruitment and training. Origins of lawyers who settle into different legal careers show recruitment patterns similar to those of house-staff physicians. In law, only 16 percent of the men in independent practice and small firms came from top law schools, and in medicine the same portion, only 16 percent of our sample of house-staff physicians in the small, nonaffiliated hospitals have gone through the top schools in medicine.[5] In medicine, the tendency toward bifurcation provides the possibility for planning training sequences that make use of the different directions and different personal dispositions and abilities, and that can foster excellence within each direction.

Theresa Rogers suggests something of the plight of the people in university hospitals whose career plans do not conform to the modal pattern.[6] Only 31 percent of the future general practitioners training in university hospitals felt their clinical judgment surpassed that of attending physicians at least several times. But in the nonaffiliated hospitals, where they are not so clearly atypical in career plan, 63 percent said their own clinical judgment surpassed that of attending physicians "several" or "many times." Some of the difference may simply reflect differences in the competency of attending staffs in the two kinds of hospitals. But beyond that, the feeling that a house-staff member has about his own competency compared with that of senior physicians may influence his conception of himself and his relationship to medicine in as yet unspecified ways. One can argue that the young physician could come too soon to assurance that he knows better than his seniors, can become insensitive to his own inadequacies. At the other extreme, the low-status student from a low-ranking school who somehow joins a "proud company" in an affiliated hospital could become too unsure, or he might become a disheartened isolate in medicine.

The internship and residency experience can affirm and reinforce the direction that a medical student has already taken. But when program and student are oriented to distinctly different ways of life in medicine, the resulting incompatibility may produce disaffection with training and something undesirable in later practice. The hospital and program that proves intellectually challenging and lively for one intern may be experienced as a threatening, uncomfortable, and alien environment by another.

In a visit to five hospitals within one community that had a medical school I interviewed a number of interns and residents who had had experience in both of the two university-affiliated hospitals. Some had also worked as medical students in one of the three community hospitals, and they seemed to have some definite ideas about the character of the different hospitals. They also suggested that certain types of medical students were drawn to each of these hospitals. The matching experience of the five hospitals shows that the two university-affiliated hospitals have done consistently well in attracting interns. Of the two, Hospital A is nearest to the medical school, and in this and some other attributes it is somewhat similar to the University Hospital of this study. Its house-staff members speak of "high morale," and of the benefits of having time to consider many aspects of a case.

The other affiliated hospital, B, is owned by the county, and it is across town from the medical school complex. This hospital incorporates some attributes of both Community and University Hospital, and it has its own unique quality. A resident's advice expressed a theme in this hospital, that is, it is assumed that everyone will be doing a lot of reading in the medical literature, but the resident will be willing to bring literature to the intern so the intern will not lose a moment of what is most important —the patient. The resident said: "Get your resident to go to the library for you and bring back references you want. If you leave the floor, you will just find that you're missing so much.

You can go, but it is really so important to be here that it seems too bad to leave the floor. The emphasis is really on learning, learning the most you can and you only learn really at the bedside." Voluntary sacrifice may increase loyalty to a group or to some of the group's goals and values, and contribute to group morale.[7] Many members of this hospital's house staff had a wide choice of internships, and they chose the one that offered more work and fewer physical comforts than many. Machiavelli advised, "It is in the nature of men to be as much bound by the benefits that they confer as by those they receive."[8] At least one contemporary study has found that making sacrifices for an organization can increase loyalty to it.[9]

An intern in Hospital B had gone to this town's medical school and had experience as a student in both of the affiliated hospitals. He speculated about differences between students who chose Hospital A at the university and his peers who came with him to the county hospital: "Some of my classmates who went there were just more stuffy and would probably continue through their lives in that kind of setting." This intern's perception of his own group as somehow more dedicated, more willing to go out to patient and community and, at the same time, also willing to admit uncertainty and share knowledge and responsibility is part of the ethos of Hospital B. For many able young physicians this hospital appears a congenial place to learn and to serve. But some other interns, who plan to go into practice, would not like the quality of exposure, the intellectual pace and sharing in Hospital B, and they would not like to work only with poor people. These, as two interns from Hospital C, a private community hospital, put it, "found the county hospital depressing."

The first intern I met in Hospital B asked me if I had heard about "our chart system." He and other house-staff members of Hospital B seemed proud of the system, as they were of other hospital directions. For example, in the interest of giving continuity of care, the patient is assigned a physician on the house staff and he will have the same doctor for as long as they are both in the hospital. Interns in this hospital go to considerable efforts to set appointments in the outpatient clinic at special times so their own patient doesn't have to wait. At the orientation breakfast, the new interns are given a small black notebook and are told it is for the intern to write down pertinent information about his patients so he will have it available should one phone for help. These house-staff members seemed much more actively involved with the family and work situations of their patients than house staff at University Hospital appeared to be.

The differences between the three community hospitals in the same town illustrate the fact that no two community hospitals are alike. Some elements that are often associated with affiliation can exist without the fact of affiliation—and with similar effect. For example, the one unaffiliated hospital in the city that is most successful in recruiting interns and residents is Hospital E, where all attending physicians are there full time. This is a hospital that also has exceptional building and educational facilities for its house staff. We have quoted one intern in this hospital who said, "There is something to be said for practicing medicine in pleasant surroundings."

Hospital E, although without university affiliation, is also somewhat like University Hospital in its specialization, research, and education interests, and in the national repute of some of its senior physicians. But it is different from University Hospital in that it relates much more closely to physicians in private practice outside the hospital. Hospital E offers an active continuing educational program, and it has established mechanisms to attend to the local practitioner who refers a patient for special diagnostic work-up or therapy. The member of the attending staff who is in charge of a case during hospitalization writes his discharge summary partly *for* the referring physician. The patient is thus clearly returned to the care of the physician outside the hospital and the system of referrals between colleagues is confirmed. This contrasts with the patterns in some university hospitals of the country where private practitioners outside the teaching hospitals and without staff appointments are essentially excluded from meaningful exchange with people inside the teaching center. In this, Community Hospital E may offer promise for the nature of specialized service that some community hospitals can contribute toward continuing education of local practitioners in their communities.

A small event suggests the viability of Hospital E's relationship with men in private practice. When I wrote to arrange for interviews and observation in this hospital, the prompt and affirmative reply added a reminder of the dates of the American Medical Association meetings, implying that some of the attending staff would be away from the hospital a few days. The dates of the meetings were apparently somewhat less relevant in the other hospitals, for no one else mentioned this time conflict.

Community hospitals C and D are also without formal affiliation, although some of the attending physicians in these hospitals are also known and respected in the city's medical school. These two community hospitals offer their interns contacts for future practice and the possibility of becoming attending physicians there. These hospitals also include some admirable clinician role-models and they have strong programs within certain specialties. Hospital C and D also offer flexibility. The "late bloomer" who might otherwise be shunted prematurely into a specialty has a chance to move more to the pace of his own stage of development. One intern at Hospital C had not decided on a specialty and found that he could work out a program tailored to his needs. A resident said, "It was just what I needed." Another resident said, "The ideal thing about this program is that you are not just there, you can work out a program . . . squeeze the sponge wherever the water flows . . . I have just had a month at Massachusetts General in Boston."

One intern at Hospital D, who was a graduate of the city's medical school, compared his experience with that of affiliated Hospital A (where he served as a senior medical student). "It was like going from hell to heaven when I came here." Another said, "We did not have the rapport with the teaching staff there at the university hospital . . . This has been a friendly internship . . . you are not the low man here. When I rotated through a service at the University Hospital A, I always ended up making one enemy. I have not made one here." The perception of this intern that "we did not have rapport" raises the fact of different responses to, and perception of, a single environment. For other students, that same place—University Hospital A—was just the right environment. It was stimulating and rewarding. A chief resident at Hospital A had said, "I have been delighted to be here. I enjoy seeing patients and being able to think about them for a time and then come back to see them." His career plans included teaching. He liked the contemplative investigation of the university setting that an action-oriented individualist in a community hospital could find frustrating.

We have seen that schools differ in the portion of recruits who stood high in some of the nation's best schools. "From the standpoint of the medical school, it is reasonable to maintain as high academic standards as possible. However, a problem exists in that medical schools have no other goals for their students which are so clearly defined and measurable as high academic performance."[10] The fact is that hospitals, like medical schools, can also vary in the personality types they attract as well as in the career plans that characterize their recruits. There is evidence that medical schools differ even in the proportion of students who score high on the authoritarian scale. Moreover, students who score higher on authoritarianism, tend more often to select general practice, while the proportion of those selecting internal medicine and psychiatry decreases. The findings of Coker, Greenberg, and Kosa in their survey of over 2,500 medical students in eight schools suggest, "that authoritarianism is correlated with a preference for general practice and a rejection of internal medicine and psychiatry, while Machiavellianism is correlated with a preference for psychiatry and rejection of general practice."[11] As the promising matter of personality and selective recruitment is pursued in more detail and considered in relation to real variations in hospital learning environments, more efficient use of different hospital environments and different types of students should follow.

Presently, those students whose personality, stage of development, and future plans are compatible with the teaching hospital probably have the best chances for an internship position that will suit them. In turn their rewarding experiences in housestaff training also provide force toward positive and consistent influence within the medical profession.[12] These students who are moved along the university-educational continuum with encouragement and advice about which specific programs would be most compatible with their inclinations have a double advantage. They are most likely to have stimulated the interest of their faculty role models, and these faculty physicians often know in some detail about programs in the nation's teaching hospitals. Thus, chances are good that student and hospital will be well matched. Then such students are also usually backed up with letters of introduction and recommendations to other university hospitals. They have wide choice of internships.

The student who has not prospered in the affiliated hospital where he worked as a student may not receive much help toward finding the best hospital for his personality and career plans. This is partly because faculty members may be less interested in him and partly because faculty may be less familiar with the rich variety of programs in hospitals without medical school affiliation. As Richard Saunders points out in his report on training programs in twenty-seven hospitals, faculy members often know too little about other programs, particularly those in nonuniversity hospitals.[13]

An attending physician in one community hospital volunteered, "The University has ducked its responsibilities in a real sense. It casts its boys out and doesn't want to do anything about them if they are not University material. In so doing, it has not helped to upgrade the health care of the public." Possibly related to this, doctors in general practice do express a relatively high rate of dissatisfaction with their medical education. At least one study found a positive association between encouragement given to students by faculties and the class rank of the student. Students toward the bottom of the class who receive least attention "may be the ones most in need of encouragement" and thoughtful placement.[14]

As Joshua Fishman urged, "It may be of some help, for a while at least, to de-emphasize prediction per se and to consider how different kinds of students make different kinds of uses of different kinds of college environments."[15]

Consistency and Variety

University Hospital attracts men of similar background and experience more consistently than Community Hospital. Interns at University Hospital typically come from the major medical schools of the United States. Five of the eighteen straight medical interns one year were from the hospital's own affiliated school, with the others from Harvard, the University of Virginia, Vanderbilt, Duke, Boston University, and Yale. Community Hospital interns come from a wide spread of medical schools and a number of countries. In one year, for example, one house-staff member had been through a small southern medical school; two were from large metropolitan schools; several interns arrived from Switzerland; one from Germany; one from Scotland; and two from England.

Differences in backgrounds, experience, and training of the Community Hospital staff as they arrive is suggested by one resident's report of "almost violent disagreements within the house-staff about which procedures should be used." The variety of reasons that interns offered when asked why they selected Community Hospital for internship also suggests diversity: "Plenty of green space without cars for my kids"; "potential for practice in the community"; "pleasant atmosphere." One intern said he had decided he would not try to go to a university-affiliated medical school when he discovered that his wife was pregnant. He named an out-of-state university-affiliated hospital as the place he had first hoped to go. Several Community Hospital interns reported that this had not been their first choice for internship. A few foreign interns arrived with some misconceptions about the hospital. A resident from Switzerland reported that he and two friends had decided on this internship after they had talked with a fellow countryman who was enthusiastic about his training at Community Hospital. "We were surprised when we got here that this hospital had no affiliation. It hadn't occurred to us that a hospital with an internship training program would not have such affiliation." In spite of their surprise, the Swiss house-staff members said they were glad they had come.

Wide variation of background among the house-staff members

characterizes the small, nonaffiliated hospitals of the country. In the nationwide sample of interns and residents 95 percent in the large, nonaffiliated hospitals gave the United States as their country of citizenship; less than 70 percent of the respondents in small, nonaffiliated hospitals indicated they were citizens of this nation. A much larger portion of the members of large, affiliated hospitals said their parents had been born in the United States, and were college educated, and as we have seen, their medical training has generally been in the more prestigeful schools.

House-staff members in different hospitals are, of course, aware of this factor in their environment. Eighty-eight percent of the University Hospital residents thought that most of their staff colleagues came from the nation's top medical schools. At Community Hospital, not one of the house-staff members checked "most" of their fellow staff members as having been to "top medical schools." This too, is like the pattern of the national sample. Over 56 percent of the respondents in large, affiliated hospitals, but only 16 percent of those in small, nonaffiliated hospitals reported that they came from schools ranked either "top" or "second."

In recruiting from the top schools, University Hospital has two advantages. There is self-selection by those applicants who consider themselves fit for an academic career.[16] The hospital can then select from an abundance of the best applicants. In contrast, Community Hospital generally gets the applicants who have not ranked at the top of their medical school classes. In addition, the limited supply restricts the choice that Community Hospital physicians have in selecting for interns who will fit.

The relatively homogeneous specialty groups of interns and residents at University Hospital provide the basis for house-staff consensus on a number of issues.[17] Whether through selection, emulation, or group impact, house-staff members in each of four specialties at University Hospital were observed talking to patients in the same manner they had seen their chief use, and some even employed the stethoscope in the same way.

Small groups with members who share similar backgrounds and values are generally the best equipped for effective cooperative efforts.[18] Thus, at University Hospital where team work is stressed, the composition of the team is often the kind that is most likely to be productive and to reaffirm teamwork as an ideal in modern medicine.

The Community Hospital intern may sometimes miss the personal comfort, reassurance, and comradeship of a group of peers who share his perspectives. But he indicates that he benefits from the variety his hospital provides. American-trained housestaff members at Community Hospital consistently mentioned diversity of approaches they found in their environment as an advantage. One said, "You get to see 100 approaches." Another volunteered he liked "being able to select whose advice to ask." Individuals with personal reasons for coming to Community Hospital do have a good opportunity to select the physician whose interests and abilities seem compatible with their own goals.

Though diversity can serve individual interests, it can also create problems for the hospital. The intern at Community Hospital is exposed to many different approaches and he says he benefits from that. The organization also benefits—through the individual initiative that it fosters—and administration and the medical staff of Community Hospital point to this aspect of their hospital with considerable pride. Yet the intern at times complains of lack of cooperation within the house staff. Executives in the organization sometimes also express concern over "lack of group spirit in the house staff."

Attracting people for diverse reasons and from a variety of cultural and socioeconomic backgrounds, and then encouraging each member to make his own way and establish his own contacts with individual attendings makes Community Hospital liable to some special problems of competition within the house staff. This is paradoxical, for precisely the hospitals that seem to have the most relaxed and friendly atmosphere may also have most problems with house-staff members who don't get along with each other, and who compete in ways that can be destructive of group cohesiveness. A collection of people of diverse backgrounds and goals in an organization that encourages individual initiative is unlikely to form into a close-knit high morale group.

As Barnard put it: "The most intangible and subtle of incentives (for full cooperation) is that which I have called the condition of communion . . . It is the feeling of personal comfort in social relations that is sometimes called solidarity, social integration, the gregarious instinct . . . it is the opportunity for comradeship, for mutual support in personal attitudes."[19]

Length of Stay

Another attribute of Community Hospital that reduces its chances to develop close-knit house-staff groups is the relatively short time its trainees expect to work together. Most of them are there only for a year.[20] When one plans to stay beyond a year, it is most often because he hopes to move into practice in the community. For this goal, gaining the approval of an individual attending physician is more useful than establishing good relations with fellow house-staff members.

In contrast, University Hospital with its full, graduated residency program, has longer to "make its mark" on house-staff members. Beyond that, the intern's plan or hope to stay through extended training may encourage him to try to get along with his fellow workers with whom he may have to work for several more years.

Some University Hospital house-staff members even repeat residency years after they have fulfilled their specialty requirements, and a few stay on for research fellowships. Value commitments of teaching and research—that no amount of knowledge is enough—stimulate the desire to prolong training. The hospital's graduated training program in several specialties and research possibilities make extended training in the environment possible. The intern who joins a house-staff in this context is likely to be aware that he can gain from getting along with fellow interns and residents, and he has good chances to find house-staff members in his specialty at University Hospital who share his interests and "talk his language."

Osler Peterson's study of ninety physicians in general practice and in internal medicine points up the significance of length of training: "After age 35 . . . the quality of medical training does not appear to be as significant as its length in influencing subsequent performance."[21] It is not just that the doctor may learn more as he accepts more years of training before practice. It is also that the decision to stay implies certain commitments. Then the group of physicians left in training at each successive stage becomes increasingly homogenous, increasingly strengthened and identified with standards of practice implied in long, specialized training.

The environment has a greater chance for influence on the individual the longer he voluntarily exposes himself to it. This, plus relative homogeneity of background and of medical specialty interest, escalates influence toward still more consensus within specialty at University Hospital. David Caplovitz, in his study of medical students, found that "as they move from one stage of training to another, they become more fully indoctrinated into the value system of the medical school. Thus, when asked which faculty members they especially admire, the more advanced they are, the more likely it is that students will indicate an instructor who has not yet, but who will soon, receive public recognition of the esteem in which he is held by his colleagues on the faculty."[22]

University Hospital house-staff members within each specialty could be observed sharing impressions and coming to *group* estimates of an attending physician, a resident, and others. These members were also more uniform in attitudes and behavior around chart work than were Community Hospital people on the house staff. In contrast, Community Hospital interns showed wide variations in their estimates of people they worked with. One resident praised the pharmacist as a person in the hospital to whom he would often turn for advice, but his fellow intern, after admitting that the pharmacist "really knows his drugs" added, "But I do not like to see a layman in this kind of advisory capacity he assumes . . . I think (the biochemist) too, steps out of his proper role."

Extended time in the University Hospital environment also increases the probability that house-staff members will make finer distinctions when they evaluate the performance of physicians, services and facilities in their hospital. At University Hospital a second-year house-staff member said, "Of course, some attendings are better about some diseases than others, especially when you get someone like Dr. K. with a cardiology case. He can give you an awful lot. Or, Dr. G. with GI problems. This is another function of the resident—to know who the 'good people' are and let the interns know." Another resident at University Hospital said, "Depending on your impression of the attending, you will present one kind of case or another." As one group discussed a case, an intern volunteered, "You know, Dr. X. is quite an authority on tics." Speaking about laboratory work, a second-year University Hospital house-staff member said, "Counting platelets is very tricky.* You can't do one or two and be sure you are right. In reading results you even have to know *which* technician did them so you can figure the *individual* margin of error, or the test results are meaningless."

At Community Hospital, comments about physicians, as a rule, are related to more gross differences. For example, one said, "We have a few garrulous attendings who, if you . . . ask a question, will answer for an hour, cite patients they have had for years, etc. There is a good deal of variation from time to time. Sometimes you are completely on your own; at other times, if you are interested, they spend a good deal of time here."

Plans for the Near Future and Relevance of the Peer Group

The expectation of relative permanence in a setting influences behavior in subtle ways, and plans for continuing in the training position characterize many University Hospital house-staff members.[23] A first year resident at University Hospital, for example, when asked about his plans for the future, said, "I will probably continue right down the line [through graduated residency training in his specialty] although I sometimes get the feeling I should be leaving." A University Hospital intern in medicine, who had previously taken an internship in surgery and had gone through the hospital's affiliated medical school, explained he would probably spend *six more* years in the hospital as a surgical resident.

---

* A little plate or plaque; specifically a blood platelet or thrombocyte, an irregularly shaped disk containing granules but no definite nucleus or hemoglobin. These number from 200,000 to 800,000 per cubic millimeter.

Because Community Hospital offers only rotating internships, it comes as no surprise that its house-staff members have widely different plans for the next year. One year two interns said that they planned to go into general practice—one into independent practice and one into "large group practice." Two said they planned to go into radiology, and two into internal medicine. (The two who planned to go into internal medicine were only "fairly certain" of their specialty decision, and one of them was later reported as a drop-out from residency training.) Other plans included neurology, dermatology, and psychiatry. No intern specified teaching or research as his major area for work. Another year, one Community Hospital intern had started practice in the community; some others planned to settle in similar or nearby communities after residency.

In our nationwide sample of interns and residents, only 1 percent of the interns in large affiliated hospitals, but 11 percent in small, nonaffiliated hospitals reported that they did *not* plan to take a residency. Nearly one third of these interns in the community hospitals who did plan residency indicated that they did *not* plan to take their residency in their present hospital. This difference in expectations effects the degree of influence house-staff members are likely to have over each other.

The man who expects to stay with a group for several more years is usually more subject and responsive to its control than is the person who knows he will shortly go away. In such different organizations as schools, prisons, offices, and hospitals, the process of identification with the group and then later disengagement prior to moving from it can be observed. Stanton Wheeler, discussing socialization into the role of prisoner, refers to "interference" when the inmate nears his time of release. "There is evidence . . . that from the inmate's perspective, the length of time remaining to be served may be the most crucial temporal aspect. Many inmates can repeat the precise number of months, weeks, and days until their parole date arises, whereas few are equally accurate in reporting the length of time they have served." "Inmates appeared to shed the prison culture before they leave it . . . there are almost as many conforming inmates at time of release as at time of entrance into the system."[24] Interns are also accurate in the number of days or weeks left to serve, particularly when the end of internship will be followed by a move either away from the hospital, or away from training into practice.

Some breakdown of organizational or group control of members might be anticipated from the members who expect to leave soon. Whether they are prison inmates, house staff of a hospital, patients, or college students in the dormitory, as they anticipate a new role outside, approval from the old inside group becomes less salient. Both identification and control potential of the old group weakens. The movement away from the old group to some new one also influences the potential of friendship formation within the group. "Interaction increases friendship formation only in a group that is a 'going concern.' "[25] The University Hospital situation provides relatively more chances and more rewards for cooperation and friendship formation within the house staff. Community Hospital provides relatively more opportunities and impetus for identification outside the house-staff contingent. For a Community Hospital resident, a decision to stay on for another year, "had worked out very well . . . I know the doctors *in the community* much better than I did at the end of my internship."

At the Community Hospital welcoming dinner we heard attending physicians advise and encourage interns to make their own way, try to become friends with individual attending physicians, and to gain their attention. This offers encouragement for the intern and resident to try to gain favorable notice *over* his peers, rather than *from* them. Community Hospital house-staff members have many opportunities to make friends outside their own house staff. Work patterns afford the individual in the smaller hospital many chances to work directly with people in various positions throughout the hospital. Also, the Community Hospital intern and resident have free time to explore friendship possibilities outside the house staff. In addition, the intern lives on the same grounds with some members of the administrative team of the hospital, and not far from some attending physicians and other people in the hospital. He and his wife and his children may "run into" people and families of the senior staff as they move about in the suburban community.

Competition and the Social Structure

Some social structures exert pressure toward competitive behavior.[26] Community Hospital is closely identified with its community and trains recruits to take their place in it. Following this, Community Hospital interns compete for the favor of some attending physicians and for the social contacts that may prove useful for their future practice. But in addition to the fact that the competitive orientation may be communicated through the hospital's relations with the community, it is also explicitly conveyed to the interns. As an avenue for private practice, this hospital awakens, or anticipates, or strengthens the perspective intern's "business orientation" by sending him material from the local Chamber of Commerce at the time of application, and material "with the compliments of C. Savings Bank." The point here is not that the University Hospital trains its members for "the higher things in life," while Community Hospital trains them for "business." On the "selfishness-altruism" continuum, recruits in both hospitals come as everywhere else: concerned and dedicated to the well-being of the patient, semidedicated, and not very dedicated. The point is that at University Hospital, financial reward is expected to come as a consequence of status advancement within the medical academic world. But at Community Hospital, status advancement may follow either from the social esteem of the community or from financial reward.[27]

Community Hospital presents us with the paradoxical situation that a "successful" year—one in which the hospital attracted a larger number of American interns than previously —is usually followed by failure to recruit so successfully the next year. This is all the more puzzling in view of the fact that interns usually inform their medical schools about their learning experience and the general climate of their internship. If their experience is successful, one would expect that they would act as good "recruiting agents" for their hospital for the next year. However, it becomes clear why this prediction must fail if

one remembers that success in recruitment is not synonymous
with success in the quality of relationships within the house-
staff group. Quite the contrary, in the individualistic and competitive pattern through which interns at Community Hospital
must make their way, a larger number of American-trained recruits intensifies competitiveness. That is, when there are more
people vying for attention and favors from a limited few, the
pressure toward competitive exertion is greater. It follows then
that a year in which there was "poor" recruitment at Community Hospital will often be followed by one of successful
recruitment as soon as the word gets around, because the few
interns have less occasion to compete with one another. The
higher morale then leads them to write favorable reports to their
medical schools which will be an attraction for more numerous
applications the next year or two. But then, with a sizable
contingent of American-trained interns, members may feel constrained to competitive efforts and the chain is extended once
again.

Not only the personality of individuals, but also the social
conditions in which they work must be considered before the
pattern is understood. The Community Hospital resident who
said he "had it in mind to practice" in the community where
he took his internship, explained he had studied the Chamber
of Commerce brochure which the hospital had sent him, and
had looked over telephone listings of physicians before he
decided to apply for training. The hospital encourages this by
sending Chamber of Commerce material to perspective recruits
and by praising its town as an attractive place to settle. Arriving
with such plans, the intern will be motivated to push for notice
from senior attending physicians who are in a position to take
on a junior partner or otherwise give the young man an assist.
Such an intern will also be motivated to make friends in the
community. This pattern contributes to good will for the hospital and is not discouraged by hospital administration. However, from a different perspective—that of other interns—the
same behavior is less attractive. During one of the follow-up
visits to Community Hospital, the administrator expressed concern and disappointment over his present group of American-

trained interns who "would not help each other out, or cover for each other."

Some other community hospitals throughout the country seem to share the problem of fluctuating numbers of recruits.[28] One doctor referred to the phenomenon as "fibrilation through the Matching Plan." In the smaller community hospitals, where the senior staff may be quite stable, a major source of variation from year to year is the house-staff contingent itself. Thus, a chance factor of combination of personalities can have considerable effect. Beyond that there may be some optimum number of American-trained interns that will give highest odds for a good high-morale house staff in the particular hospital. If this is true, then one contributing factor in the few outstanding nonaffiliated hospitals that recruit successfully each year is the large number of full-time attending staff and residents compared to number of interns. Hospital E, which we have described earlier in this chapter, is one of these.

In the year when Community Hospital had only two interns and one resident who were American-trained, the foreign-trained group seemed cohesive. None of the foreign members planned to stay in the community for practice. All interns gathered for coffee breaks and there seemed a friendly atmosphere within the entire house staff. But the three American-trained members were free to act with relatively little competition for attention from their supervisors, the busy attending physicians who had private practices. In another year when foreign house-staff members were also in the majority, a Swiss resident said the house staff had a "fine time." Asked whether the two American-trained interns were part of the group's social activities, this resident said they were not, "They kept pretty much to themselves."

With six or more American-trained interns, there are more people on the house staff who feel pressed to assert themselves *individually* for attention. One intern who was a part of an American-trained majority one year explained that he had considered the possibility of staying in, or returning to the community for practice after residency. He added that he "believed two others also had the thought." It was almost as though these interns were so secretive that they did not directly reveal their plans for the immediate future to fellow house-staff members. Yet even the interns who expressed dissatisfaction with the morale of the house staff at the same time said that the hospital was a friendly place. The friendly atmosphere of Community Hospital thus did not contribute to a high incidence of friendship formation within the house staff.

During a year when there were only three American-trained interns at Community Hospital, no one indicated that "only a few house-staff members get along together socially." Lending support to this questionnaire response, there was no obvious evidence of friction within the intern group that year. But another year when there were six American-trained interns, several of them checked "only a few get along socially with the others." There was other evidence that year of friction within the house-staff group, and the administrator was concerned about it. When several interns and residents of one house staff became oriented to winning notice from people outside their internship group, both morale of the group and its potential for control of its own members could suffer and appeared to do so.

The small community hospitals of the country may share both the benefits and the problems of having interns who want to settle in the community. Just 1 percent of the respondents in large teaching hospitals reported that they had definite arrangements for private practice during internship; 10 percent of those in the small community hospitals said that they had made such arrangements during internship. It is possible that still others "had hopes," as the one Community Hospital intern put it, early in the year.

Still other data from our nationwide questionnaire points to differential pressures toward practice in the community of internship. Just one fifth of the respondents in large university hospitals said that they hoped eventually to have an appointment in the hospital of their internship. Twice as many respondents in the small community hospitals said that they expected to carry on their practice or work in the community where they had taken their internship.

At University Hospital, by contrast, several attributes contribute to friendship formation *within* the house staff and toward formation of viable groups of interns and residents. Friendships created during four years in the hospital's affiliated medical school often endured through continued years of training in the same hospital. One University Hospital resident explained why he found his first intern assignment particularly rewarding. "I worked with an intern I really respected . . . he was my roommate in medical school." This friendship had apparently deepened through internship in the medical service, and then later through residency.

As interns and residents were told on July 1, they were joining a "proud company." The prestige of the internship at University Hospital contributes to identification with its house-staff group. Newcomers are assured that they "belong," that they would not be there if the physicians of the proud company didn't think they could carry the tradition forward. In this context, the intern is directed to his peers as friends.

Also, as we mentioned, the large number of house-staff members at University Hospital and their separation into specialty groups offers good chances of finding some members who have common interests and backgrounds and values.[29] The member of a specialty group is not usually forced to seek friends elsewhere, because he works closely with a number of people who have similar backgrounds. Kendall observed a special case of influence from social structure on the very personal matter of friendship in one medical school:

> There is evidence in data collected at the University of Pennsylvania that, to a considerable extent, friendships are molded by external circumstances and change as these circumstances are altered. Thus, in the first and second years, student assignments on some, but not all, courses at the University of Pennsylvania are determined by their position in the alphabetical listing of their class. In the third year, alphabetical position is the sole determinant of divisions of the class into different student groups. But in the fourth year, alphabetical position is not used at all . . . Friendship patterns follow these customary practices. In the first and second years, about a fifth of the friendship-pairs are

separated by only one or two other students in the alphabetical listings of their classes; this percentage increases markedly during the third year, when alphabetical position assumes a more important role in class assignments; it declines again in the fourth year when alphabetical position is no longer a basis for grouping of students.[30]

Sharing interests and values can make work a rewarding experience.[31] One service at University Hospital held its own weekly "liver conference"—a time for relaxation and a drink before a weekend off. Wives in this specialty planned their own group activity, adding one more social reinforcement for specialization. Frequent comments suggested that house-staff members were friends as well as fellow workers.

Consistent and close interaction within specialty groups, plus the recruitment toward similarity of interest and plans to stay, add to chances that University Hospital alumni will carry with them some close human ties with fellow members in their specialty. The Captain's Chair, awarded at the end of training at University Hospital, is a kind of symbol of the extension of possible influence of the specialty training into personal life. This provides a social basis for the nationwide network of specialists, the cosmopolitan leaders in the medical profession. This network is later reinforced through specialty conventions and conferences.

Specialty interns will have frequent opportunities through the years to revitalize old friendships. Many of them will be active in the nationwide, sometimes worldwide, fabric of medical teaching and research. These are the men on the "gown" or academic side of medicine who may know more about what is going on in their specialty in a distant city than they know about events in their local community, or hospital, or medical society.

The prevalence of house-staff plans to stay through extended training at University Hospital has other implications for supervisory behavior. "Promotability" of the many potential supervisors of the intern at University Hospital, along with high prestige of teaching there, provides a balance of responsibility for interns.[32] There are more residents per intern in the larger hospital and consequently much possibility of supervision. Also, since interns expect to train several more years, reliance on a supervisor is more acceptable to them than it is to interns at Community Hospital. But balancing these deterrants to delegating responsibility to the intern, the residents who supervise interns most closely at University Hospital often expect to move up *within* the house staff. They progressively encourage the people below them in rank to take responsibility.

Toward the end of the training year at University Hospital, one can observe this process in action. The resident begins to delegate many of his present duties as he anticipates his next job. Having less time to supervise interns, he gives them more information and also more autonomy.

The men and women who come for training to University Hospital have gone through a series of selections, each tending to produce homogeneity within specialty. Sharing somewhat similar backgrounds of home and education, and expecting to have to work together for a number of years, the University Hospital intern is disposed to make friends within the house-staff group, and the group has good chances of offering its members a sense of sharing and high morale. For some of its members, the fact of choosing the longer way into specialty professional position may dispose them to feel very committed to the University Hospital emphasis on research and teaching. The typically rather long stay in the hospital further increases chances that house-staff members there will take on some commitments fostered in the hospital, in part because some of the members who "don't fit" may have dropped out.

Beyond this, the graduated residencies of the larger hospital offer the intern many supervisors who will soon be promoted within the staff. The intern has a place to go up within the house-staff group, and he also has supervisors who expect to move up within the systems. When there are enough positions available at each level to satisfy ambitions and plans of house-staff members, there is less urgency of competition within that staff. The intern is likely to see advantages of cooperation within the house staff and these advantages may outweigh potential gain from active rivalry and competition with peers. University Hospital builds a solid foundation for later specialty activities and identifications in the nation. But it does relatively little toward inducing house staff's identification with the local community and its medical practice.

Community Hospital offers its members a great deal of diversity within the training group, and interns and residents, as well as senior physicians there, seem proud of this stimulous toward individual initiative. Because interns and residents come to Community Hospital for a wide variety of reasons, many of them related to the potential advantages for their families both during internship and later toward practice in the community, the smaller hospital sets the stage for competition once it receives more than a very small number of American-trained interns. Having a somewhat limited basis of exchange when they arrive, the interns may look around to form friends and gain approval from senior physicians and people in the community. Less motivated to move up within the house-staff group through graduated residency, the intern can see that he has more to gain from winning approval over his peers rather than from them. In this system, a relatively small portion of American interns seems to make for high degree of satisfaction by the individual, and a successful year of recruitment breeds an element of disappointment and discontent with the intern experience.

IV | Social Networks

Work in Community Hospital directs the intern's attention to the attending physicians who function successfully within the hospital and out in the community. Many of the other people the intern works with at Community Hospital also have important roles and responsibilities out in the community. The intern who follows the pattern of engagement with the town may come to feel allegiance to his hospital and its community at the sacrifice of feelings of solidarity with his peers. He has many opportunities to see what private practice would be like. In contrast, the people of University Hospital have other roles that provide them with opportunities to teach and conduct research, and to learn whether they might like such work. Several attributes of the University Hospital puts the older man—the attending physician with a practice—at some disadvantage. At the same time, house-staff members within each specialty are placed together in conditions that make for solidarity and sharing within the house-staff specialty group at University Hospital.

Outlook at Community Hospital

The eight connected buildings of Community Hospital spread into their immediate neighborhood of homes just as personal connections in this hospital spread out into its local community. A swarm of private cars hovers in parking lots and along the sides of tree-lined driveways. These automobiles arrive, wait for brief intervals or many hours, and then depart throughout day and night—carrying physicians, families of patients, administrative workers, nurses, and volunteers to and from their individual extrahospital responsibilities. The personal lives of Community Hospital practitioners are not as isolated from their professional pursuits as the lives of professionals at University Hospital. The administrator's child may come into his father's office from his nearby home to remind him it is past time to come home for dinner. There are many occasions for people in the hospital to carry thoughts of their hospital responsibilities into the community, and for people from the community to carry their outside commitments into the hospital.

Community Hospital's significance to its local town comes into sharper focus when hospital figures are compared with its 100,000 community population.[1] Roughly, one person in seventy-seven could be related to the hospital in some "active capacity" from full-time employee to "consulting" doctors and dentists and volunteer workers. A number of women in the community take the hospital as an important focus for their social and volunteer activity. A local club for retired businessmen provided elderly gentlemen as volunteers to operate the main elevator.[2]

Community Hospital has been the major hospital in its neighborhood for over fifty years. Since the community is small compared to the metropolitan area of University Hospital, a large share of the people in the area have been in Community Hospital as newborns, patients, visitors, or workers. Community Hospital affairs tend to be available to its local community for negative or positive sanction, as University Hospital affairs tend to be available to its medical school for sanction.

Only one out of every seventeen physicians associated with Community Hospital worked there full time, compared with more than one out of two physicians who were full time in University Hospital.

Community Hospital had three full-time pathologists, three radiologists, twelve house-staff members, and a total of 272 affiliated physicians and dentists. Although the hospital is essential to many physicians in the course of their private practice, very few are on salary in Community Hospital.

The ratio of part-time nurses also suggests a multitude of

ties between Community Hospital and its town. At one time, nearly 85 percent of the hospital's 150 nurses were working part-time. Many of them are married and have their roots in the community. This contrasts with the nursing contingent at University Hospital where only about 10 percent were on part-time status. The director of nursing at University Hospital regretfully reported that suburban hospitals had an advantage in attracting nurses who would return to work after their children were in school.

Extraprofessional roles of interns are also differently patterned in the two hospitals. A smaller portion of University Hospital interns than Community Hospital interns are women. Of eighteen interns on the medical service at University Hospital in 1957-58, only one was female. But of the ten interns at Community Hospital in this same time period, four were female. One of these was reported to be pregnant, and one had an infant. This distribution of females in the two house-staff programs may reflect any or a combination of factors: recruitment policies of hospitals that have their choice of many applicants, or the recommendation patterns of professors in medical schools, or perhaps even the desire of women for some of the amenities that some community hospitals offer.

Fewer of the University Hospital house-staff members were married. At University Hospital in 1957-58, one third of all the house-staff members, including the older advanced residents, were single.[3] Only one of the interns at Community Hospital was single. Compared to Community Hospital, University Hospital has a smaller portion of professionals who have major extraprofessional statuses that might present serious challenge to the priority of learning, teaching, and house-staff duties.

Community Hospital staff members marry earlier. Some are poorer and need a wife's support. There is more extra-house-staff pressure on such interns, who tend to be more oriented to personal career, building a practice, meeting people who can help, and securing income for the type of living they desire. Thus, private interests and community interests may intrude more often in Community Hospital. The staff at University is more (though not exclusively) oriented toward University Hospital-Medical School interests: teaching, research, service. Their interest can be more concentrated in their medical career.

The intern who has a wife may enjoy benefits from flexibility and informal patterns at Community Hospital that would be absent at University Hospital. For example, the smaller hospital demonstrates greater tolerance for individual arrangements that take into consideration the intern's obligations to his family. Work schedules, living arrangements, the date he starts his internship, and occasionally, the need to earn extra money above his intern stipend are more often mentioned as legitimate reasons for administrative decisions.

Community Hospital's emphasis on individual arrangements and on flexibility, while made possible by its relatively small size, may be made necessary by the dominance of combined roles that subject many people to extrahospital pressures and expectations.

The hospital admission policy offers an example of articulation between the expectations of hospital and community. At Community Hospital the intern on admitting duty is allowed to meet the patient's and the community's need for admission without regard for the teaching potential of the case, and there is some evidence that the interns and attending physicians in this hospital think of such an admission policy as best in serving teaching needs of interns.[4] Ideas about what constitutes good teaching for the house staff help Community Hospital to function acceptably in its environment. At the same time, the hospital helps its incoming interns and residents in their adjustment to expectations about their extraprofessional life as well as about their new hospital duties.

The large corporation that encourages its executives in local offices to "settle into" local communities where they are sent—buy a home, join a local golf club, and become active in local voluntary associations—can improve chances of articulation between plant and community. In a similar way, Community Hospital, by recruiting interns and residents who may wish to develop ties in the community through their families, and through their aspirations for later practice there, can encourage attitudes and norms in its house staff that do not do violence to community expectations.[5]

Personal ties between organizations and the community can also create pressure on some organizational goals.[6] For example, refinements of teaching and research are of relatively less immediate interest to the local community than are the more visible goals of service to patients and their satisfaction. Yet the hospital's administrators and physicians who care about the training program must maintain the quality of teaching. Each year the Council of Medical Education and Hospitals must give its approval of internship and residency programs. Although a successful training program and a good reputation in academic medicine does bring qualified recruits who will contribute medical service, this cause and effect is not directly visible to the community. Thus, the personal ties between hospital and community facilitate achievement of some hospital goals, but perhaps most often those goals that lay community leaders can best understand and accept. At University Hospital, the same mechanisms operate, but in the direction of articulation between hospital and medical school.

Outlook at University Hospital

At University Hospital, care of patients is part of the academic enterprise. It is given open recognition through conferring a medical school rank to all members of the staff, even to residents. In this situation, the expectations and potential sanctions of the medical school gain salience over those which come from the administration of the hospital or the nursing service.

All chiefs of service are full professors in the medical school. The director of the central laboratories for the hospital wears two additional hats: one, that of attending pathologist for the hospital, and another, that of associate professor of pathology for the university. Many full-time physicians of professorial rank in the medical school serve as attending physicians who work with the house-staff members. In turn, the interns and residents work with clinical clerks from the medical school at some time during the year. In the medical-school bulletin, residents from the major services are included as "assistants," following the roster of the ranks of professors and instructors. From intern to chief of service, everyone acts as teacher and sometimes as researcher, not only in addition to, but also in his very capacity of the patients' physician.

The fact that the senior physicians with most prestige at University Hospital hold university appointments not only contributes to the quality of training, it also gives authority and weight to the combination of teaching students and caring for patients. The presence of medical students on hospital wards provides house-staff members with many opportunities for teaching, both formally and informally.[7] Through the day, informal exchanges—with medical students, with professors, and other house-staff members—are often facilitated by means of teaching. Intelligent questions and extended discussions in response are valued not only for the resultant learning, but also as a means of opening a conversation. The "good question" also can serve as a socially valued entree for an intern. By a good question, he shows that he belongs, for he searches after knowledge and he admits his own uncertainty. All these opportunities to teach—even in informal exchanges—provide the avenue for developing abilities and inclinations for teaching at University Hospital. The environments which provide such opportunities to recruit and train as well as try skills develop professional staff for medical schools.

The intern and resident can get to know people who teach and learn first-hand about their lives. University Hospital also provides the intern and resident many possibilities of being noticed by senior colleagues who can act as mentors for the future, and these early experiences as a teacher can also awaken in the house-staff member some taste for the personal rewards available in the teaching process.

A professor at University Hospital praised an intern for "a beautiful job" in the presentation he had made to students that day. The intern, given a congratulatory cigar, looked very pleased while the professor described the successful "initiation": "He not only gave the history . . . but he also ran down the parasitology . . . He did my whole lecture. I didn't have to do a thing . . . Some of the students came up to me afterwards and said they thought that it was a most interesting lecture." For having successfully performed as teacher, the intern was the center of favorable attention for an afternoon.

The intern or resident who has opportunities and rewards for teaching can identify with concerns over problems confronting academicians rather than with the problems of private practitioners. It is no surprise to see that house-staff members at University Hospital are more disposed to plan to teach some after they complete training than are Community Hospital members. The term, "teaching privileges," conveys an attitude found in many University Hospitals. Nationwide, more than 14 percent of our American-trained respondents in closely affiliated hospitals but just 2 percent of the ones in nonaffiliated hospitals indicated "teaching or research plus specialty" as a part of their future plans.

More important, training fashions opportunities as well as plans for later success. It seems reasonable to assume that trainees in Community Hospital who say they hope to go into teaching will be less likely to make it than will their colleagues at University Hospital. One Community Hospital intern, midway in his training year, said he would like to teach either full or part time. He did take a residency at an affiliated hospital the following year, but was reported to have dropped out.

In another large hospital with a close university affiliation, a medical student illustrated his yen to teach. He had been invited to discuss nursing from the medical student's perspective. When student nurses asked him how he thought nursing students should act in order to work better with medical students, he emphasized, "show more curiosity," "ask more questions," "let the student explain procedures." In other words, he invited them to let him serve as a teacher. His response was a surprise to nurses who had assumed that medical students wanted more "help" and cooperation from nurses and nursing students.

To one intern at University Hospital, "being an attending *meant* giving much time to teaching. He mentioned the financial sacrifice it would entail, then said, "I would love to be an attending. I think it is the best way to keep up with what is developing in medicine . . . I would certainly look on being an attending as more of a privilege than a chore." When he was asked what he meant by "a good attending physician" he said, "Someone who is able to stimulate further your thinking about a case and offer concrete examples to the best articles about a particular kind of case." Now, some years later, this intern is a faculty member in another university hospital and he is recipient of an award to extend teaching of behavioral science in the medical school.

As a number of interns and residents at University Hospital suggested, the occasions when house-staff members fulfill some teaching responsibility may also stimulate them to "keep up with" the literature. "Teaching keeps you on your toes."

At University Hospital, the opportunity to perform the task, the rewards forthcoming from senior colleagues, and the expectations emanating from younger trainees, all combine to fashion the self-image of the young physician as a future member of the academy. When clinical clerks look to the intern or resident for an informed answer, he may be particularly motivated to fulfill the expectation to "know" and to be up-to-date.

The Attending Physician at Community Hospital

At Community Hospital the attending physician tends to control access to patients. For interns who hope to practice in the community, this control projects into the future. As the administrator told the new interns, "You will be given experience in proportion to your interest. When you are in obstetrics, if you are slovenly and lazy . . . you will get mighty few deliveries to do." Interns and residents who develop skills in communicating easily with patients and their families, who learn from a senior how to take a history "without seeming rushed," and who act with assurance may attract the interest of an attending physician with a good practice.

But it is not only the attending physician's importance as a source of future referrals and advice that makes him such an important person in Community Hospital. The social structure of medical care in Community Hospital puts an individual physician in the limelight of daily medical events. The intern there joins an individual physician to move along his own itinerary to see patients. This pattern increases the chances for an intern to attach himself to an attending physician of his choice. Moreover, the Community Hospital intern does not have a conflict of allegiance between the senior whom he wants to admire and his age peers who make a claim for his loyalty and attention.

The norms and values of Community Hospital are unequivocally represented by the attending physician, who stresses care of patients over teaching and research, and effective action and initiative over the more leisurely questioning contemplation. Nor are these norms put into question by collective and symbolic appearances of groups of medical students who move with their professors from the affiliated medical school. In the Community Hospital climate, the house staff can be unambiguously impressed by a senior's ability to predict outcome of cases, to take a history quickly, to direct a course of action with dispatch, to calm an anxious patient, to manage family distress smoothly. The intern can grant the attending physician the claim of authority based on experience, on his acquaintance with particular families in the community, his familiarity with the hospital, and his long-standing record of successful performance. In effect, the able attending physician at Community Hospital experiences comparatively little challenge to his position of role model for the young practice-oriented interns and residents.

Our nationwide survey offers corroborating evidence of the relative advantage the attending physicians have in the non-affiliated hospitals. Fify-four percent of the respondents in the smaller, nonaffiliated hospitals chose an attending physician as the man they "most admired." In contrast, 37 percent of the respondents in large, university-affiliated hospitals selected an attending physician as the person they most admired. The resident was more often chosen in the university hospitals. Some of this difference may reflect the larger number of residents to chose from in the large teaching hospitals. On the other hand, it should be remembered that the university hospitals do attract some of the nation's most distinguished medical people as attending physicians—many of national reputation.

At Community Hospital, both the attending physician and the trainees recognize the importance of the attending physician for the learning experiences of interns. It will be remembered that at the orientation dinner at Community Hospital, attending physicians advised the incoming house staff to "get to know attendings," to "become friends as well as pupils." And correlatively, a resident at that hospital expressed his satisfaction after the first year by explaining, "I know the doctors in the community much better [now]." This is a far cry from the injunction, "Let's not set out to trap them (attending physicians)," which we remember from an orientation meeting at University Hospital.

Reference Groups at Community Hospital

The administrative people in Community Hospital are more active in several areas of the intern's life and they see more of interns throughout the year than was true at University Hospital.

The offices of the Community Hospital administrator are centrally located on the corridor leading to the medical records room and the hospital's single medical library. As the intern goes to the library or the record room where he dictates his reports on newly admitted patients, he usually passes by the administrative offices where the doors are always open. The administrator said, "I think we do, as a matter fact, probably get to know the house staff better and work more closely with them than we would if we were part of a university hospital." The administrative secretary, in talking about former interns of Community Hospital, seemed to know a great deal about them—where they had come from, whom they had married, where they were now, and where they planned to be in permanent practice.[8] Interns and residents had, through the years, picked up their checks from this office and often stopped to chat as they did so.

We have seen that the social structure of Community Hospital offers little opportunity for solidarity among American interns. Therefore, house-staff members need other people to act as mediators between their present and future status and between their professional and personal needs. Other people—often attending physicians or laymen—are available to answer the need. The attending physician looms large as a role model for the future career of the intern at Community Hospital. Administrative people there are important as mediators between the intern's hospital life and life in the community.

House-staff members at Community Hospital also have more opportunities to meet people in the community, either through activities in voluntary associations or through moonlighting activities for which there is more time and more acceptability here than at University Hospital. The practice of taking on some other work to fill out the intern's or resident's income should be studied. There is wide variation, informally, between hospitals about moonlighting, and the variance, I believe, is not accounted for by objective need of the individual staff member. For example, in one community hospital, an advanced resident was reported to have been a "moonlight doctor" in order to pay for his swimming pool. In some community hospitals the house staff takes on the cooperative responsibility of seeing that the emergency room in another hospital is always manned at night. Senior staff in some hospitals with regulations against moonlighting tend to look away when house-staff members take on some jobs; for example, doing examinations for insurance companies. But the same hospital may be more vigilant against moonlighting when it takes place in another hospital's emergency room.

Community Hospital trainees have access to a wider variety of social relations than do their peer-group-oriented colleagues at University Hospital. Paradoxically, the very complexity of the social network available in the community hospital is also a source of frustration. At University Hospital in-group solidarity and dependence on the specialty group tends to encourage trainees to compare themselves and the rewards they obtain with other interns. At Community Hospital the intern has a wider variety of persons to compare himself with, and the rewards of many of these people will exceed his own in one aspect or another.

Community Hospital trainees rarely compare themselves with

their counterparts at University Hospital. They hardly know them or the details of their work. One intern at Community Hospital who had previously been a clerk at University Hospital did say, "The intern works less here." An intern may wish vicariously to raise his professional status by stating, as one did, "We have enough time for leisure so we can be human beings." Generally, however, the interns evaluate their own work load, pay, and social relations by using people above them in rank. Thus, their perceptions are colored less by objective conditions than by their comparisons with people outside the house-staff group. The Community Hospital interns are also influenced by expectations raised in the hospital's emphasis on "friendliness" or "getting to know the attendings." Against these heightened expectations, they "did not have enough time for reading," "did not see much of the attendings."[9]

Community Hospital interns seem more prone than University Hospital interns to express disappointment over not being taken into the bosom of the attending physician's social life. In the smaller hospital where many people do seem to have friends at work, the intern may feel more "deprived" by lack of friendships in the hospital than he would if he were part of a larger hospital where less is said about "friendliness." One intern mentioned his disappointment at not seeing attending physicians socially. Asked whether he had ever been in the home of an attending physician, he first said, "no." Later and in another context, he reported that for a part of the year there had been regular informal journal meetings in the homes of surgeons, and he had attended these.

An unanticipated consequence of the "relaxed atmosphere" is that people *expect* more individual arrangements and more gestures of friendship from attending physicians and others.[10]

The Inner Circle: A Frame of Reference at University Hospital
When interns at University Hospital measure how well they are doing, how much they know, and how satisfied they are with their training, they often use the young research-and-learning oriented physicians—residents and fellows—as a frame of reference.[11] Just as one group is put in a good light by the

conditions in an organization, another group can be put in an unfavorable light. When this happens, the norms of the people in disfavor become relevant because they are assumed to be bad; "negative reference group" refers to the phenomenon of looking to a group for what *not* to do. Which groups are favored or not so favored can then influence the inclinations and perceptions of interns, and help fashion their perspectives and actions.

The value commitments and the social structure of the larger, affiliated hospital tend to draw favorable attention to the younger men in specialty groups, the residents. Rapid technological change and scientific advance give the young man who has just completed full-time study a distinct advantage. He knows all about the latest advances while the older man is behind. Teaching the sciences today thus demands more of the teacher. First, he does not have the social advantage that a store of vast, arcane knowledge would bring; some portion of what he has learned has been superseded.[12] Second, he stirs discontent with present knowledge: he must teach his students to doubt, not believe, to question, not accept.[13] In succeeding, such a teacher then sets the stage for the challenge of his own position. Where cumulative knowledge and related enterprises of teaching and research are emphasized, the physicians who are in the hospital full time, doing research and teaching, have an advantage over those who are "only in practice."

House-staff members at University Hospital can have a feeling of being at the leading edge of knowledge in their specialties. They see more patients with some rare diseases than physicians in practice usually do. When the field of comparison is the latest information about *unusual* problems, the house-staff physicians hold a distinct advantage over the attending physicians in practice.

Other attributes of the social structure of University Hospital also contribute to chances that the house-staff member there will look to his peer-group of relatively young men for standards and that he will identify with them. The intern or resident at University Hospital is in close interaction with members of his specialty group during many of his waking hours.

Often exposed to group pressures, he is relatively protected against potentially effective demands from outside. Chances are good that he and his specialty group will be able to stand together and to believe, as the saying goes, "that the brothers are all valiant and the sisters are all beautiful." A corollary of this in-group solidarity is an occasional tendency to be critical of those outside; for example, of the relatively older man with a practice.

Still another element of the University Hospital structure puts the younger and full-time members of the hospital in a favorable light. The patterns of work within a specialty tend to place the resident in the center of communications regarding complex diagnostic problems. Indeed, the scheduled group activity that characterizes the work of each specialty group at University Hospital does more than increase chances for strong and enduring identification with peers in a medical specialty. It also seems to buttress formal communication lines and the prestige system of the house staff, and this, in turn, increases the tendency for interns to look to residents for assistance, advice, and apparently also to use these relatively younger men as role models.

For the most part, the people to whom the intern is supposed to turn for help are also the most convenient people to ask. They accompany him on morning rounds, review charts in the nursing station, go with him and a fellow intern to look over X-rays. At night, either the chief resident or the assistant chief resident is on duty, and a cardiology resident is assigned to take night calls. On his ward, the assistant resident is the person immediately responsible to assist and advise, and is often there much of the day.

Herbert Simon observed: "In the organizational hierarchy, the superior ordinarily enjoys, by virtue of his position, the same advantage of information over his subordinate. The extent to which this advantage is real, and the extent to which it is mythical, may depend in large part upon the design of the lines of communication in the organization. The superior who possesses such advantages of information will have much less occasion to invoke the formal sanction of authority than the superior whose subordinates are in a better situation than he, from the standpoint of information, to make the decision."[14]

In his orientation talk on the first day of internship, one chief of service said, "Preserve a very precious system—graduated specialization. Call the assistant resident, the resident, and only then the attending." In daily experience these people are often present or near the intern in this order. They are also likely to have first-hand information about the intern's patient in this same order.

Residents who are given formal responsibility for guidance are on the ward, and they can give immediate suggestions out of their own first-hand information. At the same time, they can draw on their up-to-date knowledge in their area of specialization. The resident's central position in communication for task-solving also contributes to the tendency among house-staff members to impute superior knowledge and skill and leadership ability to residents, occasionally, to the disadvantage of those attending physicians who are not full time in the hospital.[15]

In the preceding chapter we discussed self-ratings by house-staff members when they were asked to compare their clinical judgment with that of attending physicians. We noted that the interns and residents who planned to go into general practice were in a minority in the affiliated hospitals and that relatively few of them felt confident in their own clinical judgment when they compared themselves with attending physicians. But in these same affiliated hospitals more of the men who planned some teaching and/or research indicated confidence in their own competence. Conversely, more of the general-practice-oriented interns who were in "their own element" in nonaffiliated hospitals indicated feelings of confidence in their clinical judgment compared to attending physicians. Now we are concerned with a different problem—the selection of people that house-staff members use when they evaluate themselves.

In our nationwide sample, house-staff members in the large, affiliated hospitals reported that they used residents more often than they used attending physicians—when comparing how good their medical performance was. As Table 3 shows, this was true in the large affiliated hospitals even when the skill was something which might be enhanced through experience and maturity: "ability to cope with social and emotional problems of patients."

TABLE 3

PEOPLE WITH WHOM HOUSE-STAFF MEMBERS COMPARE THEMSELVES WHEN THEY EVALUATE SPECIFIC PERFORMANCE IN THE LARGE, CLOSELY AFFILIATED HOSPITALS (N = 961 RESPONDENTS)

The people respondents used for comparison	Performance area of comparisons				
	Diagnostic ability	Ability to cope with social and emotional problems of patients	Medical knowledge	Technical skills	Your standards of medical care
Interns	13%	11%	16%	16%	8%
Residents	50%	45%	48%	57%	34%
Chief of service	13%	8%	8%	9%	21%
Attending physicians in private practice	14%	28%	16%	11%	19%
Teachers in medical school	8%	6%	11%	6%	16%

Source: "Codebook: Study of Internships and Residencies, Nationwide Study of Hospitals," Bureau of Applied Social Research, Columbia University, February 1961.

The situation was reversed in the small, unaffiliated hospitals (see Table 4). Figures 3 and 4 depict the tendency for house-staff members of both types of hospitals to compare themselves relatively most with residents when they evaluate how well they do with technical skills. In both kinds of hospitals, residents are referred to least in considerations of standards of medical care. But, here as with each area, residents are referred to by a larger portion of respondents in the large university hospitals than they are in the small unaffiliated hospitals.

The Old Man and the In-Group

In University Hospital and similar affiliated hospitals, an interesting role reversal occurs between teacher and student. A resident in a large, university-affiliated hospital described a weekly conference in his hospital as "offering the attending a chance to learn . . . and a chance to catch up on what is go-

TABLE 4
PEOPLE WITH WHOM HOUSE-STAFF MEMBERS COMPARE THEMSELVES WHEN THEY
EVALUATE SPECIFIC PERFORMANCE IN THE SMALL, UNAFFILIATED
HOSPITALS (N = 360 RESPONDENTS)

The people respondents used for comparison	Performance area of comparisons				
	Diagnostic ability	Ability to cope with social and emotional problems of patients	Medical knowledge	Technical skills	Your standards of medical care
Interns	16%	17%	21%	23%	10%
Residents	29%	28%	31%	37%	22%
Chief of service	10%	6%	8%	7%	12%
Attending physicians in private practice	34%	42%	27%	27%	40%
Teachers in medical school	8%	4%	10%	3%	13%

Source: "Codebook: Study of Internships and Residencies, Nationwide Study of Hospitals," Bureau of Applied Social Research, Columbia University, February 1961.

ing on." One University Hospital resident said, "We tend to look on them [attendings] as less informed and less up-to-date than we are and we might be rough in our judgment of them. But I think this attitude does keep the attending on his toes. It is very good experience being an attending here." An intern said, "He frequently learns more from you than you from him." A resident said, "The intern is more likely to have been doing more discussing and more reading and be more up-to-date than the attendings, and so he may know more about a particular problem than the attending." Another resident here said, "I do not think there is any other field where the younger men are so critical of older men. There is a premium on new ideas." A closer look at attitudes of house-staff members at Community Hospital suggests that what this University Hospital resident observed may occur more often in research and teaching-oriented medicine.

In a questionnaire comparing house-staff knowledge and skills with those of attending physicians with whom they had worked none of the University Hospital interns and residents checked that house staff were "not as good" in "knowledge of current

Fig. 3. Percentage of house-staff members who compare themselves with residents when they evaluate their own performance in different areas.

Performance area of comparisons

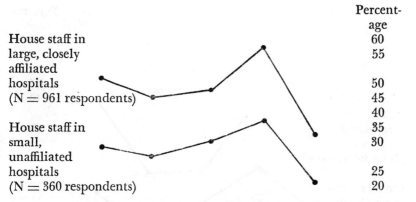

	Diag-nostic ability	Ability to cope with so-cial and emo-tional prob-lems of patients	Medical knowl-edge	Tech-nical skills	Your standards of medi-cal care	Percent-age
						60
House staff in						55
large, closely						
affiliated						
hospitals						50
(N = 961 respondents)						45
						40
House staff in						35
small,						30
unaffiliated						
hospitals						25
(N = 360 respondents)						20

Source: "Codebook: Study of Internships and Residencies, Nation-wide Study of Hospitals," Bureau of Applied Social Research, Columbia University, February 1961.

medical literature" and none checked that the house staff were "not as good" with "familiarity with action of newest drugs" compared with attending physicians. This contrasts with Community Hospital where 90 percent of the house-staff members checked to indicate that house-staff members were "not as good" in "knowledge of current medical literature" and half of them checked "not as good" with "familiarity with action of newest drugs."

Over a wide range of attributes, house-staff members at Community Hospital gave attending physicians higher ratings in

*Fig. 4. Percentage of house-staff members who compare themselves
with attendings when they evaluate their own
performance in different areas.*

Performance area of comparisons

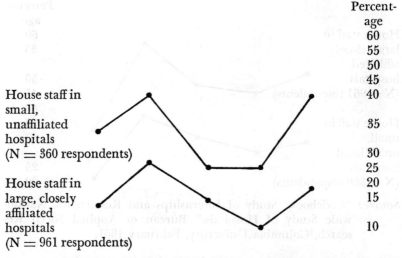

	Ability to cope with social and emotional problems of patients	Medical knowledge	Technical skills	Your standards of medical care
Diagnostic ability				

	Percentage
	60
	55
	50
	45
House staff in small, unaffiliated hospitals (N = 360 respondents)	40
	35
	30
	25
House staff in large, closely affiliated hospitals (N = 961 respondents)	20
	15
	10

Source: "Codebook: Study of Internships and Residencies, Nationwide Study of Hospitals," Bureau of Applied Social Research, Columbia University, February 1961.

comparison with themselves than did house-staff members at
University Hospital. There is no reason to believe that attending physicians who teach at University Hospital are less knowledgeable and up-to-date than those at Community Hospital.[16]
Differences in comparative ratings reflect not only the house-
staff's high expectations at University Hospital, but also the
hospital's emphasis on being up-to-date.

At University Hospital the fellow *house-staff members* are often cited as offering "a great deal" to the learning experience of intern and resident. When University Hospital respondents answered the questionnaire item, "How much do you feel you have learned this year from each of the following?", one out of every five indicated he learned "a great deal" from interns. At Community Hospital, *no one* indicated he learned "a great deal" from interns.

Still other factors cast favorable attention toward the house staff, often to the disadvantage of a potential reference group —the senior physician at University Hospital. The older man at the larger hospital often meets with a group of house-staff members who have had opportunities to develop some of their own group expectations and norms.[17] He is an outsider to the group. The group can stand in judgment of him and it sometimes does.

An attending physician at this hospital suggested that senior physicians may sense that house-staff members can be "ahead" of older physicians and reported that some may be apprehensive about confronting the house-staff group. "One man who is a full professor here . . . would call up the night before he was going to come in to find out what patients were going to be presented, just so he could read up on the problem." This possible adjustment to the house-staff group's expectations may keep the attending physician on this toes, but if senior physicians in practice are induced to reinforce, rather than temper, house-staff's tendency toward low evaluation of what some clinicians can teach, there may also be an unfortunate loss in teaching.

The "outside" physician in practice may have valuable experience on how patients respond emotionally to some procedures, about how to calm the anxious family of a patient, about ways to increase chances that a patient will follow necessary medical orders. But the senior physician in such an environment may not readily volunteer such information, may not bring up the subject of agencies in the community that can assist a patient or his family, may not be prone to insist on attention to the total situation of a patient. Ways the senior physician has learned to get significant aspects of a patient's history in minimum time without seeming brusque, or how to handle problem patients in an office practice—may be listened to with less interest in this environment and may be *offered* less often than at Community Hospital. The attending physician at University Hospital may be induced to respond to house-staff group informal pressure toward *their* definition of what is important to discuss. In this sense, the University Hospital attending physician could at times be moved to offer the kind of teaching he is comparatively less well qualified to give, sacrificing potentially useful, though at times more homely insights that are the product of years of practice.

The chief of service in another university-affiliated hospital said, "The house staff sometimes complains that attendings learn from them rather than vice versa. I think this is because the house staff doesn't appreciate just what the attending can bring to them." In medicine, as well as in any field, the student and teacher may disagree about what should be learned. There is never any guarantee that the student necessarily knows best, no matter how vocal or sure he becomes.

A former house-staff member of University Hospital said, "The fellow who grows up in the medical-school hospital gets the idea that no one knows anything but the people in his hospital . . . or in a *few* other places like his. When we got patients referred to us by other doctors (outside) . . . very little attention was paid to *anything* the referring doctor had said, though he may have known the patients months or years." Occasional jokes among house-staff groups about the way some attending physicians on private services handled chart work may even suggest that house-staff members at University Hospital sometimes put some "outsiders" in private practice in the position of a negative reference group. The term "LMD" (local medical doctor) is seldom used as a flattering term in the setting of large, university-affiliated hospitals.

A distinction of Merton's conveys the difference in orientation of men who are fostered by the two learning environments —the local physician is associated more with Community Hospital and the cosmopolitan with University Hospital. "It appears that the cosmopolitan influential has a following because *he knows*; the local influential, because *he understands*. The one is sought out for his specialized skills and experience; the other, for his intimate appreciation of intangible but affectively significant details. The two patterns are reflected in prevalent conceptions of the difference between 'the extremely competent but impersonal medical specialist' and the 'old family doctor.' "[18]

Differences in the extent of concern with imputed expertness in the two hospitals are reflected in the rosters of attending physicians for the two hospitals. Thirty-nine of the forty-eight surgeons at University Hospital were included in the *Directory of Medical Specialists and Diplomates* certified by the American Board of Surgery. Community Hospital had sixteen surgeons on its roster that year (not including consultants and courtesy staff). Seven of them were Diplomates at the time. Physicians in each hospital appeared to be concerned with formal qualifications. (The Community Hospital administrator mentioned that all the attending physicians active in the hospital are "board eligible.") But the degree of interest in the more formal qualifications and reliance on such, as well as the hospital's ability to demand the qualifications, do vary between hospitals.

When they were asked about their basis for selection of an internship, thirteen out of sixteen house-staff members at University Hospital from one medical school indicated that "quality of house staff" had been of "great importance" in their decision. Well over half of these respondents also attributed "great importance" to "reputation of the hospital."

The specialty groups that form in some university medical centers encourage some circulation of elites between university complexes. The cosmopolitan is used to working with others; for example, specialty consultants who may be strangers to him, but whom he knows are qualified by the fact of their position in the hospital. In this, the cosmopolitan will have a relatively easy time coping with work in a new bureaucracy. Furthermore, the network of each specialty spreads over the nation, bringing members together through meetings, symposia, site visits, specialty board examinations, circulation of faculty and students between medical school, internship, residency, and later, academic appointments. The cosmopolitan who moves across the country may have more good friends in his new academic post than he had friends in the immediate neighborhood of his hospital. The cosmopolitan way also contributes many chances for establishing a national reputation.

The tendency for the teaching and research-oriented physicians to be identified with specialty rather more than with local community and, therefore, to move a good deal, is well known. Caplow emphasizes the geographic mobility of certain ranks in the academic profession and suggests, "the higher the prestige of a department, the greater will be the tendency for its members to be oriented to the discipline rather than to the university. The important fact about what men in the major league regard as second-rate institutions is that men earn their academic reputations *within* these institutions."[19]

Corwin, in a comparison of aspirations of nurses who have taken degree programs and those who are graduates of diploma programs, suggests that similar tendencies may be found within the nursing profession. Degree programs (offered by University Hospital's affiliated school of nursing) hold higher national prestige within the profession than diploma programs (offered at Community Hospital). Corwin found that nurses who have completed their training in degree programs, though also interested in hospital promotion, care relatively more about recognition from the profession than do diploma personnel. Dipolma nurses seem less interested in teaching.[20]

The physician, full time in teaching or research and paid by a medical school is less dependent than a clinician in private practice on local acceptance and local relationships for his work and income. As Merton observes, "The separate roads to influence traveled by the locals and cosmopolitans thus help account for their diverging orientations toward the local community, with all that these orientations entail."[21] The prestige and income of full-time professors at University Hospital reflect something of their national renown in medical science. Positions in specialty organizations and academic associations, published contributions to research, and, occasionally, the physician's name associated with a therapy or a procedure, offer a powerful assist in moving up University Hospital ranks.

In a study of relationships between academic physicians and local practitioners, one professor in an affiliated hospital said, "I would point out, too, that for most university professors to survive, they must have an eye on publications in national journals, participation on national committees, and things like that." He continued, "University professors have a profound indifference to forums of concern to the community practitioners. We sent fifteen people to the Orthopedic Academy meeting, but the people won't go to the local forums." Another professor in this study provides a portrait of a physician with attitudes of the cosmopolitan: "I'm not sure about it, but I think so. I'm an outsider here. I've been here for 9 years."[22]

House-staff members in each hospital were asked whether they would prefer after ten years to "be known and respected by most physicians in [their] community," or, "be recognized among physicians as having made a specific contribution to [their] field but relatively little known in (their community)." Only one intern out of Community Hospital, but ten out of sixteen house-staff members at University Hospital preferred "potentional national recognition" within their specialty. Such orientation to the local community can encourage the physician's responsiveness to his patients. It may also at times remove him somewhat from potential influence and control by his profession.

V | From Student to Physician

Yesterday's medical student becomes tomorrow's physician by traveling a long way through the looking glass of confirming experiences and disquieting threats to his self-image as a doctor. The intern may have to act as the technically competent authority for a patient who is the age of his father, but at the same time he must learn a technique and learn competence through work with the patient. The constellation of partners with whom the intern works can make a difference both in relative smoothness of the transition from layman to doctor and the speed of it. These people who legitimately have some claim on the intern can have distinctly different, sometimes contradictory expectations for his performance.

In University Hospital the intern is often in the presence of other house-staff members and senior physicians when he sees his patients. In this role-set, this constellation of partners, the intern is twice deprived of protection for his still vulnerable self-image as doctor. His actions with the patient are often under the scrutiny of his student and faculty partners. In this setting he might hesitate to extend a gesture of acknowledgment or reassurance as a physician lest it look foolish to the doctors around him. It sometimes happens that when an intern says much to his patient while the group stands at the bedside, some two may exchange knowing glances, smile, or quip about the neophyte's fumbling efforts. Besides, in his concern over how the patient is perceiving rounds, the intern could miss something that a professor is saying about a case. In a real, though unplanned sequence, the intern's status as student, not doctor, is often confirmed in the process of teaching rounds. He moves perhaps more slowly to the feeling that he is the doctor. But as he matures, he comes to feel like a physician more through identifying with his colleagues than through his relationship with patients. He may become less subject to discomfort over the way a patient responds to him, but he is likely to stay relatively alert to approval from his colleagues.

The transition from feeling like a student to feeling like a physician is accomplished somewhat more swiftly at Community Hospital than at University Hospital. Several of the interns at Community Hospital said, "I feel more like a physician now than I would if I had gone to a teaching hospital." Several factors speed the transition, including the constellation of role partners to the intern's work in this hospital. There are fewer full-time physicians at Community Hospital and these are precisely the people who tend to relate to the intern more as student. The intern is more often alone with a patient or with patient and nurse and these people can help him to feel like he is the patient's doctor, not just a student. Also, some of the intern's work at Community Hospital includes tasks that the attending physician would otherwise have to do. In doing this work at Community Hospital, the intern serves more as the junior partner to the physician rather than as a student to teacher.

The fact that interns at Community Hospital tend to plan private practice for their near future also helps make their role as physician come alive to them. Also, the nature of medical problems most often faced in Community Hospital provides the intern relatively good opportunities to "feel like a physician." Patients are simply taken as they come. The intern sees what one attending physician referred to as "garden variety" problems. In contrast, at University Hospital, specialized services attract patients with special problems and admissions to the wards are screened in favor of challenge of the case as teaching material, and these problems are by definition not so easily solved.

This means that the intern at Community Hospital is presented with more patients whose problems are amenable to the treatment he can provide. After he learns to handle a common problem, his chances are good that he will have another opportunity soon for similar success. Mary Jean Huntington, studying the development of self-image of medical students, observes, "students who felt they handled the problems of their assigned families without difficulty showed a greater tendency to develop . . . professional self-image, even as early as the end of their first year." Where the student's ability was insufficient to meet the problem, development of self-image is probably impeded.[1]

Indeed, at Community Hospital, one of the themes that ran through the interviews with interns was their pride in ability to "cope." Frequently, this theme was accompanied by claims that they might be better able to handle emergencies than their counterparts in teaching hospitals with more prestige. Whether or not their perception is accurate, their conviction helps motivate them to undertake decisions on their own.

Physicians in Community Hospital seemed to feel that the intern could and should take on a somewhat considerably wider range of responsibilities than people at University Hospital considered appropriate. Community Hospital interns are probably right when they say they take on more responsibility than do members of the house staff of large teaching centers. Every one of the house-staff members interviewed at Community Hospital mentioned with some pride his impression that he had gained confidence through individual action, through being in situations where he is pushed to take lonely responsibility. A Community Hospital resident volunteered, "The intern arrives for his year really quite well prepared for many of his duties, though he doesn't know it. He has butterflies in his stomach, and *he can't imagine he can know enough* to handle emergencies." An attending physician at Community Hospital said, "The intern should begin to shoulder responsibilities before he goes into specialized training . . . He would return to the hospital having worked in the front lines."

One Community Hospital intern said, "In the big university hospitals they are impressed by the man who can spew forth much literature, cite chapter and verse. He may not be able to manage well when it comes right down to the situation when he is the doctor and the patient depends on him, but he sounds awfully good in a group." Attending physicians at Community Hospital at times expressed a similar perspective. One criticized what he felt was excessive protection of the intern in "some university hospitals. The intern is so protected from life's real emergencies he gets little chance to develop the kind of assurance and judgment he must have to practice mature medicine. If you start in an outlying hospital like this, you *have* to learn to apply right away what you have learned."

University Hospital interns also state they learn most when "alone with the patient," "when you are *it.*" Occasionally they complained about having someone "peering over your shoulder," or about "mother hens hovering around." One said, "Do you know how you become a doctor? By sticking your neck out, and every step you're scared."

Interns in both hospitals say they want to be "given as much responsibility as possible." But interns from the two hospitals would not agree on what is "possible," or appropriate. One University Hospital resident said, "If these people [residents and specialty residents] aren't available [to the intern], I think you might lose a lot . . . maybe it would be too hard to admit you had made such a serious mistake." A University Hospital intern expressed disapproval of rotating internships: "I think it is dangerous because *you cannot know enough to do anything* and what's worse, *you might not know enough to know you didn't know enough.*" An attending physician in one university hospital discussed the possibility that an intern who worked alone much of the time might not become aware of some of his mistakes, and could assume he was performing adequately, "a case of too much comfort with one's own inadequacies." Such cautionary comments were frequent both from attending physicians and house-staff members at University Hospital, who responded to a battery of questions about *who should* and *who does* perform nine different specific tasks. In both hospitals the intern and resident most often checked the same positions in the "who does" column as he did in the "who should" column. Thus, they seemed to indicate some sense that distribution of responsibilities to house-staff members in their own hospital was generally appropriate.[2] There were some marked differences, however, between responses in the two hospitals, indicating that the house staff at Community Hospital tended to prefer an extension of responsibilities and the staff at University Hospital preferred a limiting of responsibility. That is, when members in the smaller hospital did suggest a difference between who is responsible and who should be responsible for a task, they eliminated some *other* position than their own. Thus, they recommended narrowing of responsibility to themselves. For example, if an intern reported the intern and the resident were responsible for a task, he would be likely to drop the resident when indicating what *should* be. Attending physicians (including chief of service) were dropped seven times out of nine when house-staff members at that hospital saw a difference between what did happen and what should happen.

When University Hospital house-staff members responded to the same questions, they reported more sharing of responsibility by intern, resident, and others, and they seemed to feel this is what should be. When they indicated there should be a change, they tended to *add someone else*, or to *eliminate their own position*. Moreover, the pattern of response at University Hospital was to assign responsibilities upward, to someone with more advanced training. This is consistent with the teaching hospital's emphasis on formal qualifications and on awareness of how much more there is always to know.

The Meaning of Consultation

The University Hospital intern establishes the habit of easy and informal consultation. Peers, students, fellows, teachers are often at his side, or available for casual exchange while he reads charts in the nursing station, or moves about the hospital. The intern or resident in the teaching hospital does not have to expend much extra effort in order to consult. It is a part of the social life of his hospital and there is some evidence that he may at times not even be fully aware of the extent to which he does use his colleagues for advice, or as a kind of sounding board.

Community Hospital interns suggested that they soon noticed

in retrospect how much they *had* depended on such casual consultations while they had been clinical clerks at medical-school affiliated hospitals. One of them recalled: "The first feeling (upon arriving at Community Hospital) is a sense of loss because you are used to being in a hospital where there are three or four people standing around you all the time, [but here] . . . suddenly you are alone with the patient." This intern talked about the early weeks of his internship: "I never had any hesitance about calling for help, still you just have a different feeling when you are in a room alone with a patient than you have when you are there with another clerk or intern, and maybe a resident."

As this intern recognized, the Community Hospital intern is often more aware of *when* he is calling for help. When interns most often see patients alone there is less frequent opportunity for "disguised consultations." When he calls an attending physician at Community Hospital, the intern or resident must assume responsibility for the call. He is also responsible for which details and how much history he will report, for the attending advisor may or may not have seen the case. The resident at Community Hospital described some different reactions from attending physicians as they were awakened by an intern who called for help. "He [the intern] soon learns discrimination in when to call an attending for help. The attending indirectly teaches by his reaction to the midnight call. For example, one man on the attending staff always wants to know *all* about the patient, when he is awakened. The intern soon learns not to go rushing off to call the attending before he has checked a number of things on the patient. He learns to think through what the problem really is he is asking about."

A faculty member in an out-of-state medical-school hospital who had been trained at University Hospital, suggested some enduring effects of "growing up professionally" in an environment where collective decisions are a way of life. He suggested that at University Hospital physicians felt easy in consulting relationships but that in his present hospital they did not. "There is a great fright about consulting here. It is viewed as an admission of inadequacy to ask for advice or consultation."

The intern at University Hospital cannot go far from reminders of limits to his knowledge. He spends much of his time with people who see themselves as students and others who take pride in their teaching role. He also is not encouraged to explore for himself the individual or idiosyncratic help potential of many individuals throughout his large hospital. His organization provides him with comparatively clear and reliable clues for guidance to the proper person or position to go to for different problems.

Moreover, taking responsibility for setting a full course of action without consultation is not encouraged at University Hospital. Repeatedly, during initiation day, the intern is encouraged and admonished to ask for help. In another university hospital on the first day, medical interns were told to call their resident immediately if a patient seemed very ill. "We expect you to call." The resident's signature was required as a reinforcement for the expectation of consulting.

The availability of medical personnel and the presence of specialists and "visits," or attending physicians as consultants impresses on trainees how much there is to know and to learn— further confirmation of the student role. The fact of specialty teams also conveys the importance of making decisions with due deliberation and not too hastily. At University Hospital decisions are often arrived at on rounds by the team, headed either by a chief resident and often by visit or specialist; the "order" given by the intern thus usually follows the "recommendation" of the visit. The structure of life in the medical ward reinforces and facilitates collective deliberation rather than lonely decision.

In the smaller hospital, consultation is more an event than it is in the larger hospital where it comes naturally in the course of a day. Through its structure, University Hospital thus encourages development of one type of physician: the professional who feels responsible to his colleagues, derives gratification from their approval, and at the same time, receives a measure of protection from them.[3] Community Hospital helps the individual "entrepreneur" to develop. He is more on his own, more often has to stick his neck out, and he may do so more readily. As a clinician in his future practice he will be somewhat more dependent on the approval of the community and may seek his protection there with laymen as well as physicians, than will be true for the specialist who stays in a teaching and research setting. This pattern of obtaining gratification, protection, and help from whatever source is anticipated during the years of training in Community Hospital, where the ethos of friendly atmosphere and the social structure both encourage the intern to turn to many different sources of support. He is responsible for deciding whom to consult and he may decide not so much by title and degree as by his first-hand experience, which has informed him both of the ability and the receptivity of the persons he might ask for help.

As soon as the intern arrives at Community Hospital, he starts to hear about *individual* characteristics, idiosyncrasies, and predispositions of both attending physicians and hospital staff members. The Chief Resident may "fill him in" on the pharmacist, a charge nurse in the emergency room, the woman in the administrative office. Each of these persons has been in the hospital many years and has developed his own job in a special way as the hospital grew.

The Community Hospital intern has enough time on his own to seek out the individual attending physician. There are not so many active in the hospital but that he *can* get to know most of the "significant" ones. The fact that most attending physicians have offices outside Community Hospital means that the intern may discover that formal designations in the hospital's list of attending physicians do not consistently serve as accurate or useful guides about which physicians will be most helpful.

The chief pharmacist is a working example of individualized development of positions in the less bureaucratic hospital. He said, "In a hospital where you have attendings trained all over the map, you have 140 doctors, you have 140 different thoughts about which drugs are best for a specific thing. I can know the minute I see the attending list what drugs I will be needing to stock up on." He discussed drawbacks he saw in the formulary system—where only pharmaceuticals approved by hospital committee are stocked. (The formulary is a book that details properties and reactions of all drugs that are stocked.) "A rigid

formulary system protects . . . the intern against any consequences of trying to mix incompatibles, but he never learns
why some things can't be done, or he hasn't had the chance to
feel his way with various dosages of the same drug."

With almost 85 percent private patients, and with most physicians working outside the hospital, there is no formulary in
daily use at Community Hospital. Instead, the pharmacist gets
to know the individual attending physicians and their patterns,
and he stocks his pharmacy for them. This pattern is not unusual
in small, voluntary hospitals. One study of prescribing techniques reports, "The hospital with the longest list of . . . prescribed drugs was the smallest hospital [a voluntary one] and
did not take on the most complex medical problems."[4]

In sharp contrast, the chief pharmacist at University Hospital
described his task as much more circumscribed: "If there were
no formulary, it would mean that there would be very little
standardization of therapy, or of drug stocks in the institution,
and this would, in turn, make it much more difficult for the
house staff to gain an impression about what therapy is done in
the hospital. It makes it more difficult for the intern or resident
to avail himself of any established attitude toward medication.
A formulary implies a conservative attitude." The chief pharmacist at University Hospital emphasized "established practices"
and was concerned about exceeding his formal role and perhaps
offending physicians. He would like to be called more often and
pondered ways he could make it clear to physicians that he was
available for *them* to call for consultation and help. In contrast,
the chief pharmacist at Community Hospital does not wait to
be consulted by a doctor. He calls each intern down before the
end of the year to go over some problems of prescription writing,
such as the danger of prescribing a large quantity of barbituates
at a time.

The Community Hospital administrator, aware of the extent
to which some positions in his hospital have been subject to
personalized expansion, said, "If it weren't for Mr. X (the pharmacist who has been there for many years), the pharmacy would
be run quite differently." Expressing one aspect of his hospital's
permissive attitude toward individual arrangements, when he

was complimented on the imaginative and pleasing use of color throughout the hospital building, this administrator said, "We use the same color consultant as [University Hospital], but *here* we let him do what he wants." Here, as alsewhere at Community Hospital, the individual is less circumscribed. He is more on his own.

Intern-Nurse Relations

In Community Hospital the nurse is sometimes the most immediately available person who knows the patient as well as the hospital personnel, and she is acquainted with routine and prevailing problems. She can at times offer help without being specifically asked. Also, where most physicians have outside practices, the leadership potential for nurses seems increased. Any "credit" for leadership ability and knowledge that may fall to the position that happens to be central in communication about patients may, at times, fall to the nurse.[5]

Emphasis on personal development of roles also allows the nurse to take on more responsibility than she would in University Hospital, and it may help the intern to accept some limited advice from a nurse and to acknowledge that the nurse contributes to his learning. This does not mean that the nurse acts as a physician, or "advises" the intern as one physician to another. She simply seems to take a more active part in letting the intern know about "the way" something is usually handled in her hospital. She volunteers information more readily than her counterpart at University Hospital. Also, some attending physicians at Community Hospital, by example, encourage the intern to rely on the nurse.

As the director of nursing at Community Hospital said, "the individual attending . . . gets so he relies pretty much on certain nurses . . . he has gotten to know. He has come to trust them to call him if one of his patients is in trouble." Where attending physicians routinely have offices and practices away from the hospital, and where the hospital is not so heavily populated with doctors, the attending physician may see relatively more objective need to learn to work smoothly with nurses. Physicians in practice seem to get to know which nurses they can safely rely on for information when a patient's condition changes. Also, mature nurses tend to assume more responsibility in situations where they have been established for a long time, and Community Hospital provides an environment where the nursing staff is relatively stable, and somewhat older than nurses at University Hospital.[6]

Both the doctors and the administrator at Community Hospital confirmed the importance of the nurses. For example, nurses on emergency room duty are given explicit and repeated support for a somewhat active role in the early days of the intern's year. In an introduction to the emergency room and its procedures, we observed that the resident told all the new house-staff members they "shouldn't be embarrassed" if the nurse makes a suggestion to them. Within the several orientation sessions, the hospital administrator, the chief of the surgical department, the anesthetist, the surgical resident, and the medical resident had each specifically referred the incoming interns to nurses for some information and help. The hospital gave nurses additional backing by allowing them to hold *their own* formal orientation meeting for interns. This was in marked contrast to University Hospital's orientation meetings.

A resident at Community Hospital described the role of the charge nurse in the emergency room: "She has been there for thirteen years . . . (and is) able to offer effective assistance and support." The emergency room has a monitoring system, letting people there hear ambulance drivers in the vicinity who report on cases they are bringing in. The resident explained that the charge nurse knew the voices of most drivers and was familiar with the tendency of some to exaggerate and others to under-report. This nurse used *her judgment* about whether to call the resident or others to help the intern. When it was necessary, help was usually there before the patient arrived, without the intern having to ask for it.

An intern reported: "The crew (in the emergency room) is pretty steady, and there isn't much of a hierarchy. They just help each other. The nurse is pretty important because she has been there a long time and has handled a lot of emergencies." "Because she has been there a long time" is not the full explanation of the comparatively large significance of the nurse for the intern's learning experience in Community Hospital. Clinical experience gained over time *is* important, and tenure may reflect two-way influence between the person and his organization and thus give him particular advantages in helping a newcomer into the organization. However, the matter of which person is likely to be immediately available to give effective help in a way that is approved and that does not demand acknowledgment of a need for help, may also contribute significantly to the importance of this nurse for the intern. The charge nurse in the emergency room is *there*, and she is given explicit support in the hospital for a somewhat active role. Also, she (and some other nurses frequently mentioned as being "most helpful") seemed skilled in unobtrusive guidance that can protect the intern's image of himself as one who is "able to cope." These same nurses can be observed saying, "This is the way it is done here;" "we always . . . ," and so on, suggesting they often know hospital norms so they can protect the intern from some obvious "gaffes" in his new environment.

Toward the end of his year, another Community Hospital intern discussed nurses: "I find them very helpful, especially if you are nice to them. The nurse in the delivery room was very helpful. I think the one who was on at nighttime is a better teacher than any doctor . . . She knows what to expect . . . We have one real peach-of-a-supervisor . . . In an emergency, she would be the first to come and she could help."

A Community Hospital resident volunteered: "The nurse can teach the intern a great deal if he is willing to learn from her. This is one area where the personality of the intern can really get in his way. If he is not willing to take information or help from a nurse, he can miss a great deal . . . I will never cease to be grateful to Miss X for helping me through a couple of tight spots. And she helped me without the patient ever being aware of it." Interns, residents, and practitioners who had been through the internship at Community Hospital acknowledged, explicitly or implicitly, the importance of having nurses help "without the patient ever being aware of it."

Midway in the intern's year more than one Community Hospital house-staff member volunteered that the intern's personality—or how "nice" he was to nurses—could be an important factor in his learning experience vis-à-vis nurses. The intern's chances for very uncomfortable as well as very rewarding experiences in work with nurses are probably increased where nurses receive formal support for their individual initiative and help, and where receiving help "without the patient being aware of it" has considerable relevance. Nurses have a wide variety of informal techniques that allow them some control over the doctor, even though he has formal authority. The nurse can stick to the letter of an intern's orders, at times to his embarrassment. She can "forget" to remind him that a procedure needs to be done—until he is at dinner. She can stand by and wait for his "orders" while he flounders. The nurse's potential for control is probably greater when she has developed in a position where she does some informal teaching of the house staff, and where the intern is not backed by his own close-knit specialty group.

In both University Hospital and Community Hospital, interns and residents sometime suffer status ambiguity. As physicians, they outrank the nurse, but the nurse can know more about the hospital, the individual patient, and the particular procedure. As Rose Coser points out, "the resident's status ambiguity readily becomes the Achilles heel for an attack by the underdog. Nurses may make use of this vulnerability in the system to allay their own status anxieties and patients often emphasize or even exaggerate the resident's lack of authority."[7]

There seemed less difficulty over rank between nurse and intern at Community Hospital than would be expected with such discrepancy between formal authority and experience. Two factors may help explain this. Possibly the younger nurse, just launched into professional position at University Hospital, is more "edgy" over any threat to status than are the women at Community Hospital. Possibly, also, the younger nurses at University Hospital may take courage for overt criticism of the intern when the environment emphasizes his status as a learner.[8]

The responses to one question, "How much do you feel you

have learned this year from each of the following?," gave the house-staff members a choice: "a great deal," "a fair amount," "only a little," or "nothing at all." At Community Hospital, nurses were more often credited with contributing "a fair amount" than were interns *or* attending physicians. Nurses were mentioned as often as residents. But at University Hospital nurses were seldom credited with contributing "a fair amount." Two implications may be worth considering in situations where able nurses are somewhat excluded as a potential source of learning and information for the intern. First, the nurses are around their patients more of the day than are interns. Thus, it is at times the nurses who have most first-hand information about the social and emotional factors relevant for making decisions about a patient and his management. Second, nurses out of degree programs that stress social and emotional aspects of patient care may see more about the patient as a person. The intern could often listen to such observations to the benefit of his patient.

The Small Group in the Large Bureaucracy

The difference in size between University and Community Hospital has come up repeatedly. We know that larger size is associated with differentiation of functions, specialization, and formal communication.[9] However, this does not account for the main differences between the two hospitals. Technical and scientific development bring in their wake specialization and departmentalization independently of the size of the organization.[10] A small organization could not by itself deal with the demands of complex technical and scientific development that are characteristic of medical science. Modern medicine, with its many specialties and subspecialties, is represented by the teaching hospitals, and these are generally the hospitals with the most fully developed hierarchy and with more dependence on formal communication.

The person in a bureaucratic position holds his authority not simply by force of his personality, or through devotion from his followers, but because his position assigns that specific and limited authority to him. Should he resign or leave the position, another person with somewhat similar training and qualifications will move in and the bureau will continue to function.

Specialization, hierarchy, positions with organizationally defined responsibility and authority, and formal communication and procedures—some of the attributes of bureaucracies—are more visible and more highly developed at University Hospital than at Community Hospital.[11] Although physicians in each hospital at times looked at administrative work and formal communication as a nuisance, people at University Hospital do not seem to complain much about "ritual," "red tape," or "just work for administration."[12] One study of a mental hospital found that bureaucratic rigidities were viewed more negatively by personnel on wards where there were the *least* requirements for bureaucratic procedures. Where "staff members had less individual 'say' there was apparently less staff complaining about 'channels' and bureaucracy."[13]

Some of what at first seems an unexpected tolerance for formality is understandable because the University Hospital intern has a place, a group where informal exchange and more diffuse relationships are the norm. As long as he "belongs" in his specialty group, it protects him from some bureaucratic demands. Solidarity within one service is perhaps expressed at the same time as it is stimulated by situations that appear to place members of one specialty group in opposition to other groups and to make for formality of exchange with "them" outside the group. "They" could mean administration, the house staff in another specialty, technicians, or outside attending physicians. There were claims of territory as when house-staff members on one service were surprised and annoyed when members from another service came on their ward and "had not even called before they arrived."[14]

When the University Hospital intern and resident move outside their own groups to communicate with "them," they seem aware of stratification and also of formal channels. One resident chided an intern for having "skipped channels" when he called about a laboratory test: "Man, you go to the top, don't you? . . . Get down here with us Indians!" The intern seemed a little embarrassed that he had not called a resident and answered, "I wasn't trying to pull any international coup with this. I just thought he was the man to call."

Interns on one service draw bloods at approximately the same time in the early morning to be ready for their group's morning work rounds. If one person is late, the group usually waits. Even time for coffee may be determined by group pace. In addition, there are many scheduled conferences to account for intern time at University Hospital which also put house-staff members of one specialty together in "unavoidable relationships."[15]

As he sees his patients, reads in his specialty library, or stops to relax over coffee, the house-staff member at University Hospital is most often with fellow house-staff members and professors in his own specialty. On the medical service, the chief resident's office is reached by going through the medical library. The chief can know who spends much time reading the latest literature, and his interns and residents have chances to talk with him casually without having to make explicit their desire to see him, or without having to specify their wish to ask for help. In turn, the chief has many opportunities to keep in touch with his staff. Minor laboratories where the house-staff members can do their own routine laboratory work are adjacent to wards where the interns are assigned. Individual ward services have their own treatment, drug, and linen rooms. Thus, a medical intern at University Hospital is likely to see more of the people of several ranks in his own specialty than he sees of fellow interns in another specialty.

In surgery, one of the major services at University Hospital, the hierarchy of the house staff seems to be most highly developed. It is a truncated pyramid with sixteen surgical interns at the base; ten first-year assistant residents above them; five fourth-year assistant residents next; three first-year residents; and, finally, three second-year residents. A medical resident's perception at University Hospital was "the surgeons enter the patient's room by rank."

Operating-room assignments, posted each day, do give visible evidence of graduated tasks allocated to different ranks. Within the operating room, status differences are frequently made explicit as a well-articulated team works quickly and in close quarters under its executive head. During a major operation on a ward patient, the professor essentially carried the operation to a point of decision, then turned authority over to his second-year resident who was, in turn, assisted by one of the assistant residents. As the professor stepped back from the operation, each rank moved up to perform a more complex or significant task. Interns who had only watched from behind assistant residents who held retractors now moved in to hold these instruments.[16]

The Imprint of the Specialty Group

At University Hospital, the house-staff member is in some ways in a position similar to the college student who works and lives in a somewhat homogeneous group that is in close touch with faculty representatives. Such conditions seem to produce members whom others stereotype, perhaps indicating relatively high chances for noticeable impact where the student's time is effectively captured within a single environment and where there are many chances for interaction between students and faculty.[17] Groups with nearly exclusive access to their trainees have good potential for lasting impact on the person who joins them.

Experience in the specialty group at University Hospital resembles the time aspects as well as the interaction potential in training of military personnel and training for some religious orders, where individuals seem disposed over time to turn increasingly toward a single professional reference group. In this hospital, as in some medical schools, armed services, and in convents and seminaries, adult training is standardized, prolonged, and intense. In each, the recruit is subject to highly structured environment almost around the clock; outside contacts are limited, whether by formal regulations or by time demands. Such environments appear capable at times of producing individuals of similar attitudes and behavior, and sometimes even physical bearing, that may be obvious to the casual observer.

A study of adjustment at West Point describes an extreme of this direction of intensive socialization toward an exacting professional role. "Close supervision of the new cadet's entire waking day from reveille in the morning through meal formations to showers just before he goes to bed at night. Each inadequacy is immediately and caustically pointed out . . . the Plebe . . . is limited in his social activities, has little free time."[18] In another example, Dornbusch emphasizes the Coast Guard Academy's process of breaking the cadet's ties with the outside and limiting his possibilities for identifying with home and family by not allowing visits, either in or out, during the initiation stage.[19] James Gould Cozzens, in his novel, *Guard of Honor*, brings to life differences between army officers who had undergone West Point training and those who had not, and allows one non-West Point officer to wonder at the "simple, unlimited integrity that accepted as the law of nature such elevated concepts as the Military Academy's Duty-Honor-Country, convinced that those were the only solid goods; that everyone knew what the words meant."[20] In medicine, also, the idea of "service" and "duty" looms large, and it is articulated by demanding nearly total time from the recruit.

Some medical educators who express apprehension over what they perceive as a lessening of recruits' willingness to devote a round-the-clock attention to duties, reason that less concentrated time in training has implications for later, as well as current, attitudes. One physician expressed concern over the possible consequences of the tendency in many hospitals toward offering a fixed schedule of time on duty which allows more time off, suggesting that it might serve as ". . . a sanction of temporarily limited responsibility" of the physician for his patient.[21] It is possible that reduction of time demands and scheduled group activity, while desirable for allowing more individuality, has the unanticipated consequences of lessening certain commitments and influencing definitions of the role of the physician. The counterpart in practice for the protection of the "intern's time off" may be reduction in the ranks of physicians willing to make house calls. Salaried positions and group practice are presently adjustive mechanisms for changing definitions of time responsibilities. Here the patient has a doctor available for emergencies, but it is the doctor on duty then, not "his" doctor.

Everett Hughes asserts, "In general . . . the longer and more rigorous the period of initiation into an occupation, the more culture and technique are associated with it, and the more deeply impressed are its attitudes upon the person."[22] The occupations that succeed in instilling a sense of professional commitment seem to be those that provide centers where interaction within the professional group is controlled and enhanced, and interaction outside the agency is effectively limited by regulation, by time demands, and by physical isolation. The potential for close and continued interaction over common problems and shared goals within each specialty group at University Hospital provides opportunities for internalization of attitudes that Becker and Carper claim operate "primarily in clique and apprenticeship relations."[23]

A number of studies suggest that physical work arrangements can offer possibilities of much interaction between workers, and diminish it between workers and management. Such arrangements may contribute to a sense of work-group solidarity and identification of the self with the group and its goals.[24] The structure and climate at University Hospital helps the intern there identify with his specialty group, an identification that will be an essential element in his later professional life. He may move less quickly to confidence as a physician, and he seems to feel like a doctor in part through his relationships with other physicians. He cares about their approval. In contrast, the social structure of Community Hospital may provide the intern there with a context that allows him more immediately to feel like a doctor, and at the same time he may associate the feeling with his relationship to the patient, and he may be somewhat more sensitive to patients' evaluation of him.

VI | The Medical Chart

During their orientation meetings at both University and Community Hospital, interns were alerted to the legal implications of chart entries. In any hospital, charts are important in many ways for administration—increasingly as a point of contact with private companies and city, state, and federal agencies. Charts sometimes are basic to research on patient populations and essential for rational planning in distribution of facilities. Hospitals consult computer specialists, hoping to add efficiency to the huge enterprise of forms, and the recording, storage, and retrieval of the information they contain.[1] But at the same time, research teams complain about idiosyncratic chart entries, and it is common knowledge in medicine that charts are not everywhere treated with equal respect and attention.[2]

University Hospital and Community Hospital have similar formal expectations for the intern's performance in the area of chartwork. In both hospitals some interns expressed dislike at having to write admission work-ups on private patients for whom the intern was not actively directing therapy. There were occasional comments in each hospital about the problem of not being able to do "good" work-ups for private patients because there are so many to do in one day. The same number, six, was mentioned by at least one intern in each of the hospitals as the "large number" he might have to complete in a day. However, at Community Hospital the actual reported weekly average was higher.

In each hospital, the intern's complete report of physical

examination and medical history, "the admission work-up," forms the basis of the patient's permanent hospital record. The physician responsible for the patient then adds his orders for drugs, therapy, and diagnostic work, and enters progress notes on his patient's chart. The results of tests and diagnostic procedures, reaction to drugs and therapy, pulse rate, and temperature reading, are all recorded here. Any physician asked to consult on the case may look through the chart before seeing the patient and then add his findings, recommendations, and impressions to this vital document. When the patient is discharged, or dies, his physician is obliged to write or dictate the discharge summary to be attached to the chart and filed. In the event of a patient's readmission to the hospital, his former chart is available in the record room for reference by the house staff and by the attending physician working on the case.

Social Significance of the Chart

A hundred years ago nurses or family members who cared for a patient in his home could relay all that they thought was relevant to each other and the physician. The family doctor might carry in his head all he believed was vital to keep in mind about the patient.

By 1938 physicians were writing about proliferation of diagnostic tests and the consequence of this for chart volume. One illustrated his point with histories of two patients who had suffered similar heart disease and had been treated in the same hospital but thirty years apart. The entire written record of the patient in 1908 was two and one half pages long. The patient of 1938 had a twenty-nine page record.[3] Albert Wesson noted the brevity of early charts he reviewed at Hartford hospital. For example, an admission write-up completed in the 1870's read in its entirety, "Lazy, but may prove sick."[4]

Within another twenty-five years, charts for some patients at teaching hospitals could be measured by the pound, and people were complaining about duplication and superfluous material. In the late 1960's, medical journals had turned attention to the relatively new problem of how all the material in voluminous charts could best be handled for efficient storage, communication, retrieval, and review.[5]

Charts continue to gain importance as a central reference and communication point on the patient's condition on the one hand, and on the other as a possible indicator of the physician's competence and thoroughness. With computers, chart data take on crucial importance for diagnosis and for monitoring the course of a patient's therapy. "Few marriages would appear to have had dimmer prospects of success than the one between the rigorous and highly mathematicized applications of computers and the descriptive, empirical, intuitive, and often vague practice of medicine. Yet scarcely a decade after the first tentative exploration of the use of computers in the medical sciences, they have become a vital part of many medical-center and hospital activities."[6]

The chart today stands at once as product and symbol of highly developed rational systems, specialization, and bureaucratization in medicine. It is impersonal. A dispassionate statement of a line or two can forecast death, indicate radical and maiming surgery, or signify reprieve for an anxious patient and relatives. It is part of the decision-making process in the large hospital. The omnivorous bureau demands its portion of papers, properly served with information for every patient admitted to the hospital. Interns, nurses, residents, clerks, technicians, consultants, and attending physicians alike must pay homage to the bureau by feeding facts into the proper places. File on file builds mazes to protect these documents about patients, alive and dead.[7] "Pencil-pushing" and "make-work" have negative connotations for everyone, but the demand for paper work, for going through channels can be especially paradoxical in the hospital. To the sick person awaiting admission, "What is your religion?" "Your mother's maiden name?" "Your bank?" can be particularly gauling.

Patients may be asked to detail the same information that someone else already asked. Many people write in the chart, many people carry it into the patient's room, looking at it. Then, adding to insult, the patient is not allowed to look in this document on him that seems of interest to so many others.

The physician oriented to personal relationships, house calls, and quick decisions may feel chart entries are both unnecessary and inadequate. The time and effort required to complete forms is also more directly noted in private practice where the physician's time is money and he pays for clerical and other help. Moreover, the chart can lay bare imperfections of treatment. For physicians not protected by a medical team and not drilled to live with admitted uncertainty, written acknowledgment is fraught with threats to self-esteem, and it even carries legal risks. Doctors whose data and concepts do not lend themselves to dichotomies or tidy scales and numeric entries are often restive, sometimes recalcitrant about the demands of chartwork. Recognizing this, an occasional clinician attacks the bureaucratic windmill like Don Quixote and with similar effect.

The chart is more than nuisance, more than a vestigal remain, and more than red tape. The written form is a means through which values are affirmed and articulated in the modern hospital. It is an instrument for socialization of newcomers. It can confirm the group and its medical standards. It holds together the messages and recommendations in the complex, specialized enterprise mounted on behalf of a patient. Matters that in a *Gemeinschaft* society (of which Community Hospital still has many characteristics) are accomplished through personal contact, are achieved through the chart in the large specialized hospital. The chart is a significant factor in what is being done for the patient.[8]

The form of exchanges about the patient can influence their content. The chart "is the message" in the affiliated and bureaucratic hospital. The form of the chart, even beyond its content, can influence action by making some kinds of information more visible. Knowing he will have to write it all out, and that people he respects will be reading it, the intern is encouraged to take an especially good history and do a thorough examination.

Certain classes of information about a patient are easy to communicate through the chart. Other data are difficult to put to paper, and once there could easily be misunderstood. Laboratory findings, a palpable lump, age, sex can be written in tidy sentences and they are unambiguous compared to material about a chaotic family and how this is relevant in determinations about the patient. The form of the chart—whether it demands that social and emotional problems are entered and made visible, may encourage attention toward, or away from, these areas.

In the affiliated, county-owned Hospital B, which was mentioned briefly as having particularly enthusiastic interns, the chart received special attention as a teaching instrument. Its form, as it developed in the hospital, was designed to serve as a device for medical audit to help the physician toward increased clarity and consciousness of what he is doing, and to keep him alert to what is left to be done. The intern is obliged to include a front-page list of all the patient's problems, social and emotional as well as physical. As he is able to specify problems more clearly, or as they are resolved, this is noted on the first page. As the originator of this system, Dr. Lawrence Weed noted: "At present the physician has to read the entire record (often illegible and handwritten) and then sort the data in his mind . . . He and others lose their way and problems get neglected."[9] With voluminous documents, as with people in a crowd, the individual elements can more easily slip by unnoted.[10] The table of contents to problems increases the chances that the intern will not forget about unsolved problems or, if he does, it is relatively easy for his resident or an attending to catch an oversight. Where social and emotional difficulties are routinely included in the table of contents, there may be less risk that an intern will prematurely discharge a patient to a home that will probably bring about a recurrence of the illness within weeks.

The first intern I met at Hospital B almost immediately asked, "Do you know about our chart system? . . . Charts here are problem oriented rather than diagnosis oriented. This helps us keep an open mind. We don't write a diagnosis and then try to defend it . . . This way you are always open to criticism. You have to display your line of thinking and the facts you are working with . . . Once you get used to this chart system, it is great."

In Hospital B, not only does the chartwork itself become a means of evaluating the physician, but the physician's *attitude* about this hospital's approach to the chart comes to be taken as a measure of the physician. One resident said, "I think this chart approach is fantastic . . . You can always tell how good the interns are by the way they react to the chart."

Exposing oneself for audit by writing details of progress in thinking on the chart implies significant openness and a sharing, and trust within the house staff and their teachers. It also implies that the doctors who expose their progress to easy review by their peers and their teachers will have some protection against observation by laymen. At the opposite extreme from this openness within the colleague group, a physician who is oriented to his patients and their perception of his professional image will have little impetus toward such exposure. Indeed such a physician today may see very little advantage to be gained from spending time writing charts.

Patterns of behavior around chartwork differ so from one hospital to another that newly arriving interns in several different hospitals seemed sometimes to have trouble making themselves understood when they asked for information about charts. For example, we observed earlier that to incoming interns at Community Hospital "old charts" meant those from previous admissions. But to the resident at Community Hospital it means past-due admission work-ups on present patients. The aspect of chartwork that gives administration most trouble tells something of the areas of strain between different goals in a hospital. Behavior around chartwork also gives the social scientist access to the norms that are most consistently reinforced in a hospital.

Among several areas of delinquency in house-staff behavior around chartwork, there is the common and somewhat innocuous neglect about getting around to sign charts after they have been typed. There is also the more serious delay for so long in writing an admission work-up that the patient has been discharged before it is done. There may be delay over dictating discharge summaries, and inattention to nurses notes in charts is not unusual. In some cases, the hospital is troubled about failure to record progress notes on the patient, or periodic efforts are made against notes which are so sketchy as to be meaningless.

Some difficulties that go with chartwork have to do with the opposing functions that charts sometimes serve. Clarity and precision support the communication functions of charts. For the chart to be the most effective teaching instrument, details of the physician's progress in thinking about the complexities of a case should clearly be set out, and the plans and their rationale should be specified and readily observable for consultants and colleagues and faculty to see. Only through candor can poor judgment, carelessness, or fuzzy thinking have the best possible chances of being noticed by fellow physicians and by the intern himself as he writes down the history and examination results and begins to order tests.

On the administrative side, to protect itself against legal and public attacks, the hospital needs somehow to protect its members from review by laymen. Highlighting possible oversights or negligence or error or faulty reasoning does not serve administrative goals if the chart can be remanded and then laid bare for the nonphysician to criticize or for a jury of ambivalent laymen to judge.

The deeper into the complex of medical science, teaching, and research, the more respect the chart and other records receive, and the more such records must reveal specific information for colleagues to share, study, and criticize. The farther out toward practice in the world of laymen, the less tolerable such scrutiny of details becomes and the more risk it entails. The lone practitioner could be expected to have a "who has been looking at my charts" attitude. At times, commendable protection of his patient's right to confidentiality can serve also as a screen to protect the physician's incompetence. The Community Hospital administrator did mention that only a few decades ago, some local practitioners insisted that no one be allowed to look at the charts of their patients who had been in the hospital and who were now readmitted—without specific release from the practitioner.

Hospital E, which has an active continuing education program for physicians in practice uses the discharge summary in a way that can serve continuing educational ends. As a patient is discharged from this hospital, the private practitioner who referred him is sent a discharge summary. With this visibil-

ity it was not surprising to hear an intern from this hospital
volunteer her impression of the routinely high quality of these
discharge summaries. As she said about charts in this highly
specialized colleague-oriented hospital, "The charts are all kept
together here, including the outpatient notes. Some get pretty
thick. I once had one staff man ask why I hadn't written more
progress notes. In general, the staff men write progress notes
on their patients every day. Our charts have to be up-to-date
because so many of the different staff members get involved,
and also the letters have to be written *as the* patient is discharged."

In this hospital with all attending staff members there full
time, and with the attending men responsible for writing the
discharge summary that goes out into the community, it is not
surprising to hear an intern say, "Doing chartwork on time is
not an issue."

Occasions that Turn Attention to Charts

The University Hospital intern can readily observe that many
doctors look through patients' charts—consultants from other
services, as well as the chief resident, the chief of service, assistant residents, medical students and their professors.[11] At
conferences and rounds, this part of his work will at times be observed by the group. Chartwork is also potentially visible over a
period of time, for the intern cannot legitimately go back and
eradicate an earlier diagnosis or reports of physical findings;
and in the setting where some patients return, every doctor
knows that his chartwork may be reviewed by interns and residents throughout the years. Patterned replication of the intern's chartwork during a large portion of his year implies a
degree of attention and visibility of *detail* in charts that does not
seem to exist in the hospital where charts are "reviewed" and
signed, a stack at a time, and where no second admission work
is routinely entered.

With highly visible chartwork, the intern who fails to take a
careful history or to record relevant data on his patient's chart
can start a chain of sanctions.[12] Not only his peers, or transient
medical students, but possibly the chief of service, a professor,

as well as consultants, and research teams that might be interested in the case—all may notice, and they are likely to care about what appears in the chart.

The fact that the intern spends so much time with his group at University Hospital also means that the newcomer quickly learns the expectations that fellow house-staff members hold for charts. All these full-time people are quite familiar with standards of their hospital, which means that there are relatively few instances of nondeliberate violations.[13] Group members can know about any deviation and react to it before deviance takes on the comfort of a routine. When an intern knows what is expected of him, and a fellow house-staff member observes him not living up to the expectations, whether or not disapproval is verbalized the intern may correct his ways. Tolstoy observed, "I know of nothing that can offend a man more deeply than to give him to understand that you have noticed something but do not wish to mention it."[14] These informal pressures toward maintenance of group standards can be brought to bear before the potential deviant has gone beyond caring about approval of the group.[15]

The annual influx of "new-recruits" (interns and residents and medical students) may also help to reinforce high standards for chartwork. These new arrivals at University Hospital seem to approach some areas of work with special zeal. They are among the nation's interns who are least likely to be indifferent to medical school expectations for careful and detailed attention to charts. One chief resident at University Hospital said, "Interns who have worked on (our) floors as students and medical clerks are used to doing thorough work-ups and careful histories. They sometimes err in being overly thorough, but they seldom miss anything. They are used to talking over all sorts of possibilities with the professors . . . Some of the attendings get sloppy."

The house-staff group at University Hospital, moving together much of the time, can serve as a kind of antidote when the intern or resident does get "first-hand knowledge" of some departure among senior attending physicians from the outside. While assigned to a private service, the house staff regularly reviewed charts each morning. They frequently read aloud bits of attending physicians' notes, to share and to deride the physicians' presumed inadequacy in this area. Comments such as, "the way they slop these up," "that is the profundity of the day," and "he has not made any notes on that man in . . . days!" suggest that the house staff held its own standards and judged senior physicians by them. As we have seen, the attending physicians' standing with house-staff groups at University Hospital is somewhat ambiguous. In another setting where the position of attendings is more secure and has more prestige, the residents would probably respond differently. They might be quick to point out to the "greenhorns," the interns who criticized chartwork, that they are overconforming to some medical-school expectations.

A chief resident at University Hospital said interns and residents on his service, "don't hesitate in coming to us . . . in fact they almost 'collect' such material on a doctor they feel isn't careful enough." Several house-staff members gathered to look over a chart that had come in with a newly admitted patient. As they read the chart, their derisive expressions were summarized by the resident, "Well, he [the physician who had admitted the patient and written in the chart] did not go to school here anyway!"[16] Putting their "evaluation template" over the practitioner's chart confirms the University Hospital's superiority in this area and confirms high standards in this aspect of medical work. However, the same behavior and attitudes may also interfere with two other important aspects of the physician's work. First, concern for the total patient, and the kind of material his family physician may have available to add, may get lost in the attention paid to the shortcomings of the local practitioner. Second, possibilities for productive exchange between house staff and outside clinicians are diminished.

At University Hospital, many people from many parts of the hospital may see one patient—and he may undergo different types of diagnostic tests. Rational, dependable, specific routines are required for communication about the patient. In addition, many patients at a teaching hospital where they are screened for admission, will have long medical histories and detailed notes, again directing attention to charts as a significant means of communication. Moreover, complete and prompt notes in charts may be particularly needed for patients who are included in one of the hospital's numerous research projects.

If the intern is to be able to answer most of the questions likely to be asked about his patients by professors and by peers, he will have to be familiar with past chart entries. These questions about what the charts say are asked on several "public" occasions—on morning rounds, daily work rounds, on the chief resident's rounds, on the chief-of-service's rounds, on grand rounds, and at clinical pathological conferences.

Where several different physicians typically see one patient, as they do on teaching wards at University Hospital, the need for recording actions in charts is frequently called to the intern's mind, sometimes with considerable feeling. For example, one intern, who had been absent from a floor for two hours to see his dentist, reprimanded a fellow intern who had failed to make a chart entry after seeing a patient. Upon returning to the floor, the intern had glanced through charts briefly and then stopped to see his patient to explain something to her. The patient reported "all that" had already been explained by "that other doctor." On a manifest level, the colleague had "helped" —voluntarily. However, in this setting, the assistance, because not formally registered in the chart, resulted in embarrassment for the intern who was "helped." The intern later complained to his colleague. Teamwork, with the complexities of diagnosis and care of patients, can provide frequent reminders of needs for formal communication.

It is somewhat different at Community Hospital where there is rarely more than one intern seeing a patient. Nor are there interns working with research patients whose condition more obviously requires detailed recording in charts. Moreover, they do not as frequently deal with patients who have special diagnostic problems and long medical histories, nor with so many full-time physicians around the intern who might need to know what he has just done for the patient.

Deviation that Protects Conformity

Groups of house-staff members evolve ways to protect the priority of knowing the chart and history and doing careful admission work. Expectations or regulations that could interfere with chartwork review or careful entries were sometimes overlooked by senior members of the house staff. For example, though the record room sent messages to house-staff members that they were not to take charts to their quarters for study and review, they did not always comply with the regulation, and their deviation from regulations seemed protected within the group. They occasionally exchanged jokes about their dereliction in this area. A chief resident on one service relayed the record room's admonitions, requests, and pleas to his house-staff group. However, occasional failure of the group's members to comply with this hospital regulation did not seem to be taken as a primary concern by the "relayer," and this fact lessened the impact of the messages. There are tacit agreements about priorities so that violating some rules could support adhering to others. Taking charts to his room for later review made it possible for the intern to attend first to admission work and discharge summaries and at the same time read through past entries at leisure.

Conforming to the expectation for careful, detailed, and prompt admission entries was in part possible because of some laxity in enforcing other regulations. In another university-affiliated setting, Hospital B, where chartwork received much attention, an administrator remarked that a status symbol of the house staff was possession of a duplicate key to the Xerox room. "They sometimes Xerox charts or parts of them to work with. We have to call a halt every so often if they get careless and leave anything lying around."

Many interns at University Hospital appeared routinely to put off dictating case summaries on patients who had left the hospital, in favor of keeping up with current patients, and often also in favor of doing quite thorough case summaries when they did get to them. The manner in which house-staff members volunteered the number of summaries they had yet to complete recalls observations on the use of humor about deviation from ideal standards: "Jokes not only dissolved uncertainty and self-reproach that had arisen in the past, but . . . transformed (individual deviation from standards) . . . from a private exception into a socially approved practice."[17] Thus, evasion from some regulations became patterned, and those who are not "with it" in the group's spirit will be sanctioned for overconformity.[18] During one staff meeting on a medical service, a resident exclaimed: "The record room is complaining because Bill dictated his chart too quickly!" The group seemed delighted and amused at the potential discomfort of people in the record room who apparently had misplaced a chart because of one intern's "unusual" conformity to regulation. The resident continued, "He dictated it right away after the patient had been discharged and they couldn't get the summary together with the chart. It seems this [promptness] never happened before."

Chartwork at Community Hospital

Community Hospital charts tell less of what is being done or planned for the patient than they do at University Hospital. If the intern arriving at Community Hospital is motivated to spend much time reading these charts he may soon lose interest, for charts in the smaller hospital do not often offer a fund of information about complex cases.

At the end of his first week at Community Hospital, an intern was asked what surprised or impressed him most about the hospital. He did not hesitate to say, "The histories and physicals are very brief . . . much too short. When I started, I was determined I would do every one thoroughly, but I started out behind and I never caught up. I figure the only way to manage is to make them shorter." He thought that admission work-ups would not need to be shortened if help were available from medical students. But that same day, an intern who did have the help of a student joked about chartwork in a way that suggested he too had altered expectations. He laughingly asked the student, "You took careful notes and a long history?" The student chuckled and said mockingly, "Oh, sure, full history."

The adjustment of standards for chartwork can be particularly rapid at Community Hospital where the intern can soon see examples of the allowable *lower* limits for chartwork in his new environment, and where external pressure may push toward new "adjustments."[19] The intern can see how attending physicians behave toward charts for their own patients, and how interns who have just *completed* their year at Community Hospital had done admission work-ups. The charts the new recruit sees on his first day of internship are started by interns at the *end* of their internship, the time when they may have made the greatest shortcuts in this aspect of their work.

One intern said he guessed some attendings considered most work-ups on their private patients as just an administrative formality, since they "already knew what was wrong." This intern and others came to speak of work-ups on the average private admission as "scut work" for the attending physician.

External pressures for speed may be particularly acute for the beginning intern at Community Hospital who starts out already behind. The flexible, individual arrangements at Community Hospital, which allows an intern to leave or arrive before or after July first, make the early days of internship at Community Hospital at times hectic. But even the four interns who started out with the additional help of medical students also got an early start in redefining "adequate chartwork." Although the pressure of time is real, it does not account for the alteration. Interns, as others, do what is considered important and is visible in their environment. A complementary rationale develops for the behavior "that is." One intern at Community Hospital said, "If you have come out of any medical school, you are likely to be surprised at how differently things are done than you were taught they should be done. You come out [of school] thinking each history of every patient should have three or four pages. It has never really gotten through to you that 90 per cent of the history may have no bearing on the patient's illness. It may be more a ritual . . . it is good that you have this idea in medical school because you don't have . . . enough maturity to be selective . . . I think one should learn what can be left out safely . . . Here you can learn to cut corners in ways that make sense."

Relative lack of concentrated attention to charts at Community Hospital seems consistent with considerable attention to patients' reactions to their doctors and to the hospital. To the extent that house-staff members come to care about "establishing rapport" and winning esteem of patients, chartwork, which is part of the work least visible to patients, will be the first to be postponed under time pressure. During the year, Community Hospital interns joked about "catching up" with dictation (admission histories and physicals) before Thursday so their paychecks would not be held up. Several aspects of Community Hospital contribute to this apparent "adjustment"—at the same time that they help sustain the conviction that they do "good work where it counts."

At Community Hospital the intern works throughout the year with private patients for whom he has little time or stimulus for follow-up or for checking charts. Previous charts may often be "less interesting" here compared with charts at University Hospital. This is not only due to the nature of the cases and the type of diagnostic work, but the relative lack of complexity of organization, allowing a good deal of communication to take place in an informal, personal manner.

An intern, looking over a patient's chart in the nursing station at Community Hospital, asked an attending physician, "When was this girl last in the hospital?" The attending came over and sat on a table beside the intern. "Two weeks. That reminds me, I haven't written very good notes on her . . . When I was an intern, I had a patient who had everything wrong with him. I was rushing around . . . This patient was discussed on rounds and the attending complimented me on the care the patient had gotten. Then he came back to me and said, 'These notes and this history are not very good.' I had been so busy *taking care of the patient* that I had not had time for notes." The attending suggested, first by his own lack of chart entries, then by his anecdote, that action in caring for a patient was more important than a "slap on the wrist" for inadequate chartwork. Then the attending added, somewhat later in the conversation, "Actually, the better [chart] notes that are done, the better." In this Community Hospital situation, a single house-staff member asked the attending physician about his chartwork, and the attending physician therefore had a "chance" to justify not having made notes. He recast the scene in more favorable light. As some of the house-staff members at Community Hospital stated, some attending physicians there may "seldom read" the charts they sign. The attending who signs a large stack of charts at one time, reading little or none of them, does at least implicitly approve sloppy records.

Visibility and Sanctions

A 1958 report of committee findings from a study of hospital standards cites the importance of visibility in hospital training programs. "It was the unanimous opinion of the surveyors that an internal appraisal system was most important in maintaining and elevating the quality of medical care. Even when the system was relatively ineffective, the quality of care was found to be better than where no such system existed."[20]

It is an important aspect of the experience at University Hospital that within each specialty the interns, residents, and the full-time faculty members can form groups whose members know each other, and whose actions are sufficiently visible to allow for efficient social control. These colleagues who are part of the "proud company" are motivated as they arrive to uphold medical school standards. When the intern at University Hospital fails to enter something important in a chart, the chances of others around him catching the oversight are very good. The fact that he works closely with other physicians who are full time in the hospital also means that the intern will quickly learn the norms. People can see him and correct him before he has a chance to get "set" with a bad habit, and he can see how his colleagues carry out their roles. At the same time, the groups receive some protection against visibility from laymen, and they also have the protection of some permissiveness around some aspects of chartwork. These protections contribute to making it possible for the group to press for and gain conformity in other aspects of chartwork.[21]

It is obvious that interns in any hospital will be exposed to some conflicting demands on their time and attention. There is always more to do and to read, no matter how much is done. Interns in both hospitals volunteered that they had too little time. But the different social structures and value environments of the two hospitals seem to lead toward differing orientations in the resolution of conflicts over chartwork. The three types of orienting definitions Neal Gross and his associates described were the "moral" orientation, stressing legitimacy and the *right* of others to hold their expectations; another, the "expedient" orientation to the situation, where actors sought to minimize negative sanctions, to provide best defense for themselves; and last, the "moral expedient" orientation.[22]

The house staff at University Hospital appeared to hold to their own standards for chartwork, and to criticize any outside attending physician who might fail to live up to them. This apparent readiness to attend to and to criticize chartwork appeared even on private services where interns chafed under having to do many admission work-ups in a day, and where attending physicians did not all pay much attention to charts.

A resident at University Hospital said: "The distressing thing about private service in this hospital is that they [interns] get so many patients in one day—they may work up six or eight patients . . . where they would only work up two on a pavilion [ward service] . . . they do not have time to get to know the patient or his disease and to do a really good work-up and follow through . . . you get a feeling of insecurity." Another house-staff member said: "Many patients [on private services] are entered for one problem . . . you can't check on other things . . . it leaves the intern feeling insecure." More than one said he felt "insecure" about work-ups on private services—and "insecurity" seemed to refer more to the intern's definition of what was "right" than to any fear of external sanctions from senior physicians or from administration. House-staff members at University Hospital appear to take a "moral" orientation toward charts—to see the professors' expectations for careful history-taking and chartwork as legitimate.

Indicative of two different orientations to charts, an intern at Community Hospital seemed pleased at the form some interns had worked out for themselves to facilitate more rapid and efficient history-taking. In contrast, at University Hospital, an intern expressed his disapproval of any possible limiting of history for any patient: "Some places use history forms to save time for the intern. But I don't think that makes sense. The forms have just a line or two for each item, and are designed for the normal patient. You can't write just a line or two about the chest on some patients." The man at University Hospital and many of his peers take the educator's approach to chartwork, that is, that it is "his signature and professional image to his colleagues."[23] These two interns who spoke so differently about charts were each directed toward a different life in medicine and each has pursued the direction he started in internship. The one at University Hospital is now part of the faculty of a medical school. The other is in general practice.

VII | Norms and Counternorms

Norms are the blueprints for social action—the expectations that people will act according to what is "right" and desist from behavior that is defined as "wrong" or "inappropriate." However, life is not as simple as "blueprint" implies. Norms are the creation of interaction, and the multiple goals and needs of people and groups generate not one norm for each situation but several, and they are sometimes contradictory.[1]

Merton has described examples of potential for conflict between norms within the science of medicine: "The scientist should not allow himself to be victimized by intellectual fads . . . But he must remain flexible, receptive to the promising new idea and avoid becoming ossified under the guise of responsibly maintaining intellectual traditions."[2] Also, the researcher is expected to share his findings, but premature announcements of a "breakthrough" or "cure" are decried. When medical practice is added to the picture, the number of potentially conflicting norms multiplies.

In both University Hospital and Community Hospital the environment of work tends to encourage physicians to assign different priorities to certain norms. This is never formally specified; rather, it is the result of the accumulated individual decisions, directions, and reinforcements provided in each hospital. The chart at University Hospital, for example, is highly visible to many people whom the intern respects. The norm of "doing good chartwork" is consistently reinforced. Visibility increases the chances that the intern will know in detail about the expectations for chartwork in the hospital. This aspect of his work will be exposed to sustained scrutiny, and at times will be the focus of rewarding experiences when he does well, or embarrassment if he slips up. Conditions in the hospital seem to "shore up" the intern's interest in the chart through having other people he respects perform well in this area, and through the house-staff's tendency to discount or discredit the people who might be somewhat unconcerned about chartwork.

In contrast, at Community Hospital the intern's attention is pulled to other matters, for example how the patient responds to him, and how he can manage time more efficiently by "cutting corners" and "doing good work where it counts." Priority agreements in this environment tend to favor those aspects of the intern's work that are more visible to attending physicians in private practice and to their patients. The assignments of priorities are never formally specified, and interns may or may not be aware of the evolution toward the ultimate stance they will take for their way of life in medicine. Nor are the teachers in the two environments always necessarily aware of the extent to which they further selective reinforcement of some norms at the expense of others.

Since the physician must at times face situations where two equally relevant norms conflict, he is forced to choose, by action or inaction, and his direction can have significant consequences. He cannot, at each decision point, go back over the whole route of consciously weighing the validity of each norm in the light of larger social issues and the profession—as well as in relation to himself, the particular patient, and situation. To keep the whole route open would not only subject him to intolerable stress, he could not act for trying to decide. What seems to happen is that through successive acts and experiences some special weight gets attached to certain norms—the norms that receive the most consistent reinforcement from the people whom house-staff members respect in their learning environment. The young physicians build their own way of handling dilemmas until the way becomes established. Some may ultimately become desensitized to the extent of contradiction in norms that apply to performance in one area. Some will become less acutely aware of how much choice they actually have.

Conflicts between pairs of norms are frequently made explicit in poignant life situations in the hospital, and the maturing physician is likely to have special needs for development of priorities. For example, the physician's commitments to prolong life and also to relieve suffering often come into conflict. Indeed, this is a subject that medical students and house-staff physicians frequently worry about, discuss, and debate with considerable feeling.

A few years ago mature physicians may have debated these questions less frequently once they made peace with their direction; but medical advances in treatment and in surgical procedures have reintroduced old ethical dilemmas in dramatic and publicized form.[3] The removal of a kidney from a donor for transplant may save one life at violence to another. Turning off a respirator and removing an organ can prolong one "life" at the cost of at least a few hours from another. Heroic procedures to extend life are sometimes paid for by massive emotional and physical stress in the patient and gigantic cost to his family. Without some conviction about the rightness of his priorities, without some supporting psychological mechanisms and without social support from colleagues, at least a few physicians might not have courage to persevere in their quest to extend life.

We have seen that the nature of the patient's situation generates ambivalence. He may need his physician desperately and hope for "magic" from him. At the same time, the patient hates the dependency and fears that the magical outcome will not follow. The fact that the patient is in a state of anxiety through his illness sets the stage for disappointment, and for confrontation between the patient's wishes and some norms that can contribute to excellence in the practice of medicine as well as in medical science and teaching.[4] In this context it would seem inevitable that some priority agreements would have to be forged within medicine—and given mighty support—if some norms are to survive the continuing confrontation and counter pressures from patients, who are, after all, the ultimate reason for all the effort and training.

Three norms are accepted in both Community Hospital and University Hospital but are given different priorities in the two environments: the norm of the open mind or admission of uncertainty; the norm of relay learning; and the norm of graduated specialization.

The Norm of the Open Mind

Through his training, the physician is helped and encouraged to live with uncertainty, and his training for acknowledgment of uncertainty continues longer and more effectively in some hospitals than in others. For some physicians, "Medicine is a science of uncertainty and an art of probability."[5] This is an area of stress, for in the nature of the patient's position of anxiety, possible pain, and fear, he "develops an insatiable desire for information of the kind that would be supplied by definite diagnosis and firm prognosis."[6] Training for uncertainty also generates anxiety among students. One faculty member reported, "My students are dismayed when I say to them, 'Half of what you are taught as medical students will in ten years have been shown to be wrong, and the trouble is, none of your teachers knows which half.' "[7]

Running through many conversations and conferences at University Hospital are affirmations of the norm of the open mind and acceptance of uncertainty in medical findings—a readiness to admit that no amount of knowledge is ever final. Two interns and a resident seemed to express a common value when they said, "You have to admire him for saying he doesn't know." On one service, discussion on rounds, formal and informal, offered frequent comments such as, "Can't be certain, but . . ." On grand rounds for this service, the chief of service cautioned: "You *really* could be certain that that is the reason for it?" And an attending physician challenged a resident: "Are you prepared to prove that was *the* reason?" In an interview, a resident stressed his conviction that "In medicine you can *never* say something will always be." One resident said the kind of person he admired was "Somebody who realizes he does not know everything. We all have to realize how much we do not know." Other comments at University Hospital: "If they do not admit they don't know, or they might be mistaken when they first arrive, they do in a short time." "No one seems to mind talking about his mistakes." "You can never say what something will always be; you must say it is *probably* such and such." "This hospital teaches you to be a little bit skeptical about what other people say." "When you have been doing a thing a certain way for a while, you need to stop and ask yourself if you are really right." Some negative comments carry the same message: "He sure didn't like being wrong!" "He is not forging into new discoveries or exploring." People in both University Hospital and Community Hospital appear aware that a conscientious intern or resident may be apprehensive at times. However, University Hospital seems to extend medical-school "training for uncertainty" relatively farther than does Community Hospital.[8]

In one study of 507 attending physicians at University Hospital, "only 4 per cent expressed any degree of disapproval" when they were asked how they would feel if a physician in their specialty were to admit uncertainties with respect to a diagnostic problem. "Eighty-six per cent definitely approved of admitting uncertainty when it existed."[9]

We do not know at what point physicians in each of the hospitals may become aware of limits of their certain knowledge. However, it may be that where admission of uncertainty is accepted and approved more readily—and where cases are frequently complex, and colleagues are often around to remind about uncertainty—limits to knowledge are more readily perceived. But irrespective of the actual limitations of knowledge, what is important here is the desirability that it be acknowledged over and over again and that this acknowledgment becomes one of the criteria that physicians use to judge colleague performance.

Many factors at University Hospital seem to provide some of the comfort and reassurance to interns and residents that contributes to their ability to live up to the expectation for admitting mistakes, and gaps in knowledge. The chief of one service told his house-staff members there was no one who couldn't learn something. Throughout the year, the intern and resident can hear renowned experts discussing their own uncertainty of findings. The prestige of a University Hospital internship, won over applicants from numerous schools, and occasional invidious comparison between their own performance in such areas as chartwork, and the people not "of the hospital," may also be reassuring. The house-staff member in the major teaching center sometimes seems to say, "We know enough to know when we don't know." The tendency for house-staff members to give much time and energy to pursuing problems of diagnosis—and to tell each other how much they have worked—may also give some comfort. They can say, "At least we tried very hard." The creed of limited knowledge does not give immunity to ignorance, but the University Hospital environment encourages admission of uncertainty coupled with much information about what the latest literature has to say on related problems, and what multiple diagnostic results on the case reveal and suggest. Rounds characteristically included an abundance of specific information, many references to findings, and results from extensive diagnostic work.

The possibilities at University Hospital for "disguised consultations" also provide some comfort and reassurance on behalf of uncertainty and the "open mind." Statements like, "We overlooked that," "We are not certain," take some of the onus away from the individual physician's admission of either a mistake or uncertainty. Face-saving assistance and support from the group also provides a cushion that protects high standards in high-risk areas. The intern can "stick his neck out" with a question, be reassured enough to pursue investigation and tests, in spite of counterpressure from a patient and his family.[10]

Group activity and the visibility it implies also contribute to reinforcement of the norm of the open mind by increasing the probability that the intern will be forced to awareness of some limits to his knowledge. Replication of histories and chartwork on ward patients provide his peers with ample opportunity to "call" him, should he be disposed to slip over any evidence of knowledge limits. There is always someone who may question an assumption not backed by test results.

A degree of tolerance for going around some hospital regulations confirms the priority of an open inquiring uncertainty. In ordering tests and laboratory work for patients, interns and residents presented evidence of some patterned evasion of formal regulations in favor of commitments to careful diagnostic work-ups and the norm of the open, inquiring mind. One assistant resident described how one situation was handled where the group had worked out a means of sustaining its own values by "getting around" an opposing norm in some hospital regulations. The central laboratory once had attempted to "set a limit" for diagnostic tests for each floor. The resident described how his specialty "managed" the quota: "We would go around to another floor (on the same service) and see if they had any unfilled quota and if they did, we would enter the lab request through them." Although the laboratory had set the quota at a generous maximum, the regulation did not stay in force very long. The resident explained: "The lab will think an intern is ordering tests which he doesn't need to make his diagnosis. He may just be curious about something, but really that is his privilege. He doesn't get paid much in a hospital like this, but in exchange for that he should get more lab work done . . . It is a teaching hospital . . . A few people lose their heads and do order unnecessarily, but if they learn something by it, *it doesn't bother me.*"

In University Hospital obtaining knowledge, whether or not it benefits the patient, is legitimized by the value placed on teaching and learning. In contrast, an intern at Community Hospital described having learned *not* to order as many tests as she had thought necessary when a medical student.

The questioning attitude also stimulates the intern to challenge many objective "findings." When a resident at University Hospital was asked whether he often re-ran laboratory tests when he got a positive finding, he said: "Yes, it is good practice to do that." One resident said about checking laboratory results that show abnormality: "That is the only thing to do." Other house-staff members frequently talked about their own re-runs of some laboratory tests. In the more research-oriented environment, findings were often replicated before they were accepted.

This differs markedly from the pattern in the smaller, more practice-oriented hospital, where findings were more readily accepted as accurate when they came from the laboratory. In contrast to some statements by University Hospital house-staff members about re-running test results as "the only thing to do," a Community Hospital intern said: "Heavens, no!" when she was asked whether she had results re-run, or often checked slides herself.

The tendency of some Community Hospital physicians to discourage what they refer to as "excessive preoccupation with diagnostic testing" is consistent with the practice orientation of the hospital. It is expensive for patients and time consuming for them to have many tests run, and at times also physically and emotionally taxing. Comments at Community Hospital about ordering tests are in contrast to the University Hospital resident's affirmation of the intern's "privilege" to have tests run.

The norm of uncertainty fits the scientific orientation of University Hospital and it fits the pattern of colleague orientation of physicians there. Knowledge is conditional and to be replaced. "In science, each of us knows that what he has accomplished will be antiquated in ten, twenty, fifty years. That is the fate to which science is subjected; it is the very meaning of scientific work, to which it is devoted in a quite specific sense, . . . Every scientific 'fulfillment' raises new 'questions'; it asks to be 'surpassed' and outdated. Whoever wishes to serve science has to resign himself to this fact."[11]

Innovation within science represents a special type of conformity, and may require, therefore, some special social support. The scientist is expected to investigate and introduce new findings. He must move beyond existing knowledge, providing that he satisfies the criteria of evidence and procedure. Even within proper procedure, however, the innovator may encounter some resistance from time to time.[12]

Risk is implicit in innovation and exploration. The experimenter at the very least risks being wrong, with all that may imply for his self-esteem, his personal, social, and sometimes professional and financial security. In refusing to abide by accustomed ways, the innovator in medicine carries an additional burden of risk over that of the physician who abides by accepted ways. He "sticks his neck out" beyond the already unavoidable risk of working with human life.[13]

What fellow physicians at University Hospital reward as admirable admission of uncertainty can seem less than laudable to an anxious patient and his family. Most patients would enjoy a confident assurance that their doctor knew the source of their medical problem—and had in mind the specific treatment of choice. This balm of reassurance may be an enjoyment that patients at Community Hospital receive more often than do patients on the University Hospital teaching wards.

In his advice to the young practitioner, Oliver Wendell Holmes wrote, "Let me recommend you, as far as possible, to keep your doubts to yourself, and give the patient the benefit of your decision."[14] The patient benefits from faith in the outcome and faith that his physician is very concerned, or knows for certain what to do and what will happen. The extent of benefit from the patient's trust in his doctor is repeatedly suggested in "placebo effects."[15] But the physician's education suffers when a closed mind and too much certainty replaces doubt.

It may be that some patients in teaching hospitals become socialized at least to an appearance of accepting uncertainty just as their physicians are socialized to admitting it. In case presentations in seminars for nurses in a large, university-affiliated hospital similar to University Hospital, I have been struck by the apparently accepting attitude toward uncertainty expressed by some patients who have long histories of repeated admissions to a teaching center. These are the "interesting patients," and some of them do seem to take on attitudes that complement and facilitate the physician's ability to conform to some expectations of the teaching and research center. Patients on University Hospital wards can be heard to say with some pride, "They are going to try . . . now." "*We* don't know whether this will help, but . . ." Thus, even the sector that might otherwise challenge the norm of the open mind—the patient population —sometimes offers the University Hospital intern some reassurance about the legitimacy of his commitment.

The Norm of Relay Learning

Work in any hospital provides possibilities for the exchange of newly gained information and knowledge between physicians. And most physicians are "in favor" of letting their colleagues know of some new finding or something they have learned that might be used to help another doctor's patients. The Hippocratic oath enjoins the physician to share his knowledge with other physicians. But the chances for exchange—and after that the probabilities for rewarding experience following from free exchange—seem to vary by type of hospital.

We found in our nationwide survey that 82 percent of the American-trained house-staff members in large, closely affiliated hospitals, but only 37 percent of those in small, nonaffiliated hospitals indicated "almost all" house-staff members are open and free about exchanging information. This marked difference to response in the two types of hospitals seems understandable in the light of the extent of social support for the norm of relay learning observed at University Hospital. It is not simply that the two types of hospitals recruit personality types different enough to explain the difference. Rather the structured possibilities for exchange, and after that the built-in probability for rewarding experience and for prestige to be associated with relay learning contribute to the pattern.

Both in Community Hospital and in University Hospital interns and residents did relay useful medical information to their colleagues. But the incidence of such serial learning within the house staff was apparently higher at University Hospital. In the cohesive specialty group at University Hospital, the relay of medical knowledge allows the intern or resident to display what he knows to a group of people who are interested in "latest findings," the "most recent research" and who like to consider themselves as "being up to date with the literature." It also gives the speaker a chance to try out the new-found information. A listener who is interested can be a source not only of possible admiration, he can also raise a question about applicability, limits, or the source of the information and so add another bit of knowledge. Quite the contrary if the listener is not friendly. The presentation of the gift of some newly gained knowledge could simply bring embarrassment or discomfort in return. For example, the response could be a denial of the worth of the giver, "oh didn't you know *that?*" Blau described people in one government agency he studied as frequently consulting a colleague with "whom they were friendly, to avoid rejections."[16] Not only asking for information, but also giving it makes the initiator vulnerable. The social structure that makes for cohesive groups provides a favorable environment for relay learning within those groups. In University Hospital, where numerous factors make for friendship formation within the house staff, both asking for, and giving information can be accomplished with little fear of rejection and with good chances of reward. Somewhat like the situation at University Hospital, Blau noticed that "absence of interruptions and attentive listening destroyed the doubts that continuously arose in the process of making many minor decisions . . . The admiration for the clever solution . . . increased the speaker's confidence in his partial solutions while groping for the final one . . . This pattern of explicit and disguised consultations transformed an aggregate of individuals who happened to have the same supervisor into a cohesive group."[17] At University Hospital one can notice, for example, how an intern, just returned from a lecture that his peers had missed, was encouraged, by nods, questions and expressive communication, to relay in detail what he had learned. This sharing, which is most likely to occur in a cohesive group in turn makes its own additional contribution to further group cohesiveness.

Observation of some eager exchanges of "a new finding," "the latest report," or the diagnostic results on "an interesting case" recall Shepard's description of the research scientists he studied: "Personal achievement was measured in terms of increased knowledge and skill . . . Withholding technical resources was an act of hostility, and inability to contribute was a sign of low status. A lack of interest in increasing one's technical competence was a deviation from accepted patterns of behavior. Persons . . . who were not interested in obtaining it, were socially excluded from the group . . . Technical information as the currency of the group, had properties not possessed by money."[18]

On morning rounds, during coffee-breaks, or as they gathered in the nursing station to work on patients' charts, interns and residents frequently passed along information about a report they had just read, summarized a lecture they had heard, or described a case and findings that were "unusual."

The "relay learning" appeared to flow both upwards and downwards. Thus, a professor on the wards with his medical students turned to a resident and two interns to ask what their most recent experience had been with a special problem in treatment. Or a resident asked an intern how a specific finding was interpreted in a research report the intern had read. Often such relay learning between peers appears to occur spontaneously, without a previous question.

Potential role models are encouraged to relay by explicit admonitions as well as by example. An advanced resident, who was later to become chief resident of his service, reported: "Several months ago I had a talk with Dr. X. (chief of his service) about this sort of thing and he said, 'Yes, that is the wonderful thing about medicine; we can all learn from each other.' Even the medical students sometimes give us ideas or ask us a question that starts us thinking in a new way."

The relatively good possibilities for unrequested advice and reassurance in University Hospital may sustain the intern's confidence to a point where he can act effectively in the environment where demands for his performance may at times seem impossible to satisfy, and where failure has potentially profound consequences. At one staff conference, a chief resident asked about a patient, "Who took care of her?" Several of the interns and residents smiled, one chuckled and said, "Everybody." Then the resident brought his house-staff members up-to-date with information he had about the patient who had been referred to another service, and several members of the group added their experiences and impressions of this case and her history.

The combination of hospital and medical-school responsibilities at University Hospital allows for the development of increasingly compatible definitions between the roles of teacher and physician. Sharing problems that are bound to emerge from this combination or roles, physicians can develop informal patterns that help them manage conflicts, and they can tacitly assign priorities where conflict occurs most often. When the University Hospital intern or resident joins learning, research, and teaching with treating patients, his environment provides not only rewards and encouragement, it also gives him some insulation against the full force of come contradictory demands.

Medical students at University Hospital provide a complementary direction of influence on the nature of priorities that specialty groups support. Since they are no exception to the familiar fact that new recruits tend to uphold some standards with remarkable zeal, they provide many reminders of some medical-school traditions.[19] At the same time, their status as novices leaves them free to raise stimulating questions, with good effect on medical standards. Reciprocally, the admired house-staff member tends to show sufficiently admirable performance to hold on to this rewarding position. This is how the presence of people lower in rank helps control the behavior of superiors, as when the presence of children can modify the behavior of their parents. Students take histories—on some of the same cases house-staff members work with—and pore over charts, possibly at times motivated to gain notice from a professor by questioning what an intern or resident has done, or discovering something seniors may have missed.[20]

Science and the colleague system in medicine thrive on relay learning, which demands time. But, "beset by uncertainty, attendant anxiety . . . clients come to feel that professionals unnecessarily prolong their ministration: the patient feels that he is asked to come back time and again long after necessity is really past."[21] Or the patient grows restive at having to stay in the hospital for more tests and more consultations. The differences in time perspectives between the patient and the learning-oriented physician should be explored. Hospital learning environments differ significantly in the orientation toward time they encourage, and this reflects itself in the house-staff members' time orientation.[22] Time may be visibly related to money for both the physician in private practice and for many of his private patients admitted to a hospital. While there are realistic limits on the length of stay in either setting of the two hospitals, the house-staff contingent of University Hospital is perhaps under less pressure than the Community Hospital intern to respond to the patient's desire for early discharge. Some structures are better equipped than others for relay learning. The places that have most relay learning may also be among those where the patient has trouble being heard, partly because his messages must compete with a flow of intellectually stimulating messages between colleagues.

The complexity of the medical problems of many University Hospital ward patients introduces an unanticipated factor that may facilitate house-staff concentration on the intricacies of diagnosis and on relay learning. Patients selected for a teaching ward often represent repeated admissions to this or other hospitals and therefore have already been exposed to pressure to conform to some of the hospital's expectations. On ward rounds, one resident greeted a patient as an old friend. She was one of the patients referred to by this house-staff group as "interesting," and she said she had been admitted eighteen times to the center. With repeated admissions to the ward, these patients are likely to become socialized to some aspects of the patient's role, as the University Hospital house staff defines them.[23] These patients—as did those in Renée Fox's study—used humor to manage the physical, social, and emotional dislocation they shared: " 'the intravenous' (I.V.) became an important symbol for the ward. Patients sometimes jokingly referred to F-Second as the 'Hall of I.V.' "[24]

A patient who has been in the hospital before, or who has been in for some time and enjoys attention from house-staff members, can help pull new patients toward house-staff expectations. Frequent admission and extended stay, characterize many "teaching patients" at University Hospital. This means that interns there will often deal with patients who are socialized to cooperation. Rose Coser found that patients with previous admission to a teaching hospital seemed more submissive and also appeared to help socialize other patients.[25]

One problem that occurs in all hospitals may be less frequent in the teaching hospital wards that are composed of "selected" patients. As Reader and Goss suggest: "When people first enter . . . as patients, they have rarely been explicitly informed about hospital rules or professional norms for their conduct; frequently they have only a vague idea of what to expect or what is expected of them."[26]

The fact that ward patients at University Hospital are "selected" for admission by residents may add pressure for patients to adjust to University Hospital expectations for them. In his study of referral systems, Freidson reports: "The further within this professional referral system a practice is located, the more free the practitioner is of control by clients; the patient finds that there are fewer choices he can make and that he has less control over what is done to him. Indeed, it is not unknown for the patient to be a petitioner asking to be chosen: the organizations and practitioners who stand well within the professional referral system may or may not 'take the case,' according to their judgment. The client chooses his professional services when they are in the lay referral system, but the physician chooses the patient to whom to give his services when he is in the professional referral system."[27]

Freidson studied patients in a predominantly middle-class area in New York, and he observed that the well-educated patient "is more confident and cooperative in routine situations, perhaps, but he is also more confident of his own ability to judge the physician and dispose himself accordingly. A less-educated patient may be far more manageable."[28] "The poorly educated client may also mistrust what he does not understand . . . But ignorance can also breed dependency."[29]

Ward patients, although presenting their own problems of management, are easier to deal with where the house-staff group stands behind a fellow staff member.[30] Facing a group of interns and residents, the patient is less likely to challenge the authority of the physician directly, or if he does, it is also less likely that the physician will feel threatened by the attack. Some patients, of course, pressed for definite answers from University Hospital house-staff members on their rounds. It seemed to me, however, that they did so rarely. At University Hospital and other hospitals where I have observed rounds, it is often the nurse who is left to cope with some aftereffects of the intellectual fulmination of rounds. House-staff members absorbed in discussion as they walk away from a bedside, may seldom note the emotional debris they have left in their wake.

Thus, at University Hospital the intern can be rewarded often by members of his specialty group for admitting he "doesn't know," and he is relatively protected against outside criticism. His situation recalls Charles Cooley's observation, "When the workman is more sure of his position, when he feels his fellows at his shoulder and knows that the quality of his work will be appreciated, he will have more courage and patience to be an artist. We all draw our impulse toward perfection not from vulgar opinion or from our pay, but from the approval of fellow craftsmen."[31] House-staff members at University Hospital, working alongside their colleagues in close cooperation, do repeatedly demonstrate their patience to do thorough diagnostic work. Even when they are exposed to counterpressures from patients and families, who see no reason for one more test, these doctors often persevere. They also act in concert when a senior physician appears to them to "care too much" about the layman's expectations.

One University Hospital resident spoke disapprovingly of attending physicians who "get pretty soft-hearted about treating the patient as the doctor should . . . He might see his patient feeling miserable and sick and think he should not be bothered and shouldn't have to put up with diagnostic procedures because he is already so miserable . . . You can't let your sympathy or something for the patient's family interfere with your judgment. When that happens with one of our attendings [on private service], we have to talk to him." University Hospital definitions of a "good physician" and what is "good for the patient" seem to be brought into alignment with some requirements of learning, teaching, and advancing knowledge. Thorough diagnostic work-up and the norm of the open mind are sometimes taken as necessarily good for the patient in the teaching setting.

The Norm of Graduated Specialization

The specialty groups at University Hospital, whose members are thrown into frequent and close interaction over common problems, have very good chances of coming to tacit agreements that they can sustain even in spite of counterpressures from people outside the group.[32] More cohesive groups generally have the advantage in extracting conformity from members who want acceptance.[33] With the approval of his peers, the house-staff member at University Hospital can feel the safety of numbers and of sharing responsibility in a crisis. He can be reassured by his colleagues when patients or families make excessive demands. He can get help when he is rushed, and can learn about latest findings that were reported at a conference he had to miss. He can receive a face-saving suggestion from a peer before an attending physician or the professor notice that he has missed something obvious. He can get advice without having to ask for it.[34] Daily visibility within the group allows it and its members to influence and exert pressure without appearing to be "bossy" and without having to resort to explicit sanctions.

The group also helps to insulate its members from much visibility by outsiders who do not understand some problems the physicians face.[35] The fact that interns and residents in the larger hospital are more fully exposed to observation by their specialty peers, but somewhat protected against observation from the outside, gives the specialty group the opportunity to reinforce its own expectations when they conflict with what others—for example, patients and their families—expect.

The structure of the group, its cohesion, and its formal, as well as informal, hierarchy can influence the direction priorities take.[36] The inclusion of several ranks within the cohesive specialty groups at University Hospital helps explain the nature of some priorities that emerge.[37] Seniors at University Hospital, particularly residents, are part of the group that creates the norms, and through the chain of graduated residents the full-time chief of service has relatively good chances for influence. He is often a part of the group that makes the norms and sets priorities. In touch with daily action, he has access to patterns as they develop and before they are set.[38]

The norm of specialization is also one that has its counter-norm, more prized by patients; that is, they expect that the physician will be concerned not just about their chemistry and organs, but will also care about them as people. As the patient urgently needs to be dependent on the authoritative professional, he also fears that he as a person may be rejected by the authority-figure.[39] It is in the nature of specialization that not one, but many, will work with a patient, and in this situation, the chances for the patient to feel that he has been abandoned as an individual are probably increased.

Physicians who work alone and with patients in an office practice may in a sense be more similar to Weber's politicians who deal primarily with the total situation—the "art of the possible"—than they are to scientists who must "put on the blinders" and attend only to one area.[40]

High valuation of graduated specialization, like the proud history and tradition at University Hospital, supports scientific advance. Thus an aspect of scientific advance—concentrated attention to a specific and narrow portion of a field—is made an esteemed value. This, along with relay learning, the norm of the open mind, supported by daily action in University Hospital, are brought together and given coherence in the value themes.

Though physicians everywhere in this country would agree that there is a place for specialists and specialization, they would disagree in their estimate of where that place should be defined. McKittrick observed, "Specialists are by-products of the science of medicine."[41] But specialization seems less fundamentally a by-product of dealing with patients. Specialization in medicine generally takes place first in the area of inquiry rather than in practice. It is not surprising and it is also nothing new to read of many occasions when practitioners voice disapproval of specialization when it runs contrary to the norm of total patient care.

By work and example, and by objective circumstance, graduated specialization received much support at University Hospital. After he arrives, one means for the intern or resident to manage the complex and vast and rapidly advancing science is by concentration on one special area within his specialty.[42]

Information about change in career plans of medical students in University Hospital's affiliated school, and some reports by interns and residents about their future plans, suggest the continuing influence toward specialization, teaching, and research.[43] A study of University Hospital's affiliated medical college students shows "Well over half the first-year students, but less than a fifth of those about to graduate, said that they expected to go into general practice. At the other extreme, only slightly more than a third of the beginning students, as contrasted with fully three-quarters of the graduating class, told us that they expect to practice some specialty."[44]

One chief resident at University Hospital described how he had "become interested" in problems of the liver, and another had concentrated on cardiology problems. The hospital screening of ward patients provided him with sufficient numbers of patients with some unusual problems, so he could concentrate, and he came to have a reputation in the area. Specialty, and subspecialty residency, as well as fellowship positions available in the larger hospital provide some place upward for the intern and resident to go; and increasing proficiency in one area of specialization offers opportunities for favorable notice from seniors and peers in the research atmosphere.

The situation is different at Community Hospital. The presence of a general practice resident, interns, the lack of separation of patients by specialty, and the fact that internships are rotating, rather than specialty, are among the many indicators that Community Hospital does not give the norm of specialization the high priority it receives at University Hospital. In contrast, the intern at Community Hospital has many experiences to encourage him toward a more general interest in the patient.

Often by himself when he sees patients, who are frequently articulate and knowledgeable about some social and emotional components of their illness, the Community Hospital intern may be very quickly pushed toward awareness of *these* aspects of patient care. Frequently running into people who have ties outside the hospital, there is a greater chance for the intern to hear about the extrahospital life of patients. Seeing mostly attending physicians who are in private practice, the Community Hospital intern is exposed to role models who are likely to know something about the patient's social situation. Many have known their patients for years.

The patient at Community Hospital most often sees one physician at a time and, in such a context, is more disposed to reveal what worries him. Although the University Hospital ward patient also sees his doctor alone, there are more times at the larger hospital when a *group* of physicians stand around the patient's bed. The physician alone with a patient may be most likely to notice, and to hear, what is revealed, for there is less "static" in the form of other messages being sent between physicians. The University Hospital intern works more with ward patients whose educational level is generally low. Beyond that, the medical staff members frequently do not expect these patients to know much about their condition.

Two hundred and fourteen patients in University Hospital's medical clinic were studied by a team of researchers. These patients, who represented generally low educational levels and had occupations not unlike many patients on the hospital's teaching wards, were described as participating "at an extremely low level. They seldom requested information . . . seldom requested the physician to do anything, and seldom even made a statement to direct the physician's attention to something."[45] Yet, when physicians' judgments about patients' level of knowledge were compared with the quite limited knowledge their patients actually did have, physicians underestimated their level of information. It was also found that, "Physicians who seriously underestimated patients' knowledge were less likely to discuss the illness at any length with the patients, than were the physicians who did not seriously underestimate patients' knowledge."[46]

In contrast to many ward patients, private patients may more often demand explanations, and physicians may be more disposed to offer explanations. Beyond that, chances are that the patient who expects a certain level of social etiquette and politeness may tend to elicit politeness in return—or failing to achieve it, he may comment on it. Some private patients are effective in "calling" the physician who seems to ignore them or who overlooks some social amenities. When an attending physician explained to two interns, "We have reason to doubt her accuracy about this," one private patient smiled, and then said firmly, "Doctor, I see you and I are not going to work on many cases together." The tone of the rest of the exchange between the doctors and this patient changed.

As the physician becomes more highly specialized, and as the patients fall lower on an education scale, the physician may assume that the area for discourse is reduced and he may assume that absence of questions means that the patient does not want or need more information. Beyond that, the habitual perception of possibilities for communication may at times become even more attenuated. To the extent that ward patients often are less informed and less articulate about their medical problems, and less often *request* or insist on a comprehensive medical explanation, their interns may "get used to" not giving the patient full explanations.

Response to one question on the written questionnaire suggested that house-staff members at Community Hospital who see more private patients tend to be somewhat more alert than University Hospital interns to some need for "explanations" to the patient. Half of the American-trained members of the Community Hospital staff but only less than one fourth of the University Hospital house-staff members checked they "would disapprove strongly" if a house-staff member should "fail to give a patient an explanation of his problems."

An attending physician at Community Hospital who had been trained at University Hospital mused about some differences in the two environments: "I was down there [University Hospital] for . . . years, but so far as handling patients and their families, when I came out . . . I did not know much about it at all. Some of the university hospitals are out of touch with what goes on with patients. They are so busy listening to each other that they can very easily miss what the patient is really saying."

An intern at Community Hospital mentioned attending to details of a patient's adjustment to his home situation after discharge from Community Hospital—something she said she probably would not have been doing had she stayed at the larger affiliated hospital where she had been a clinical clerk.[47]

Where interns become increasingly aware of social and emotional factors in illness, they may also be encouraged to consider psychiatry as an area of specialty for them. Daniel Funkenstein's studies of trends in recruitment to and through medical schools suggest a possibility that should not be overlooked: "An accelerating trend in recent years is that many of the students with the characteristics of clinicians, who entered medical school planning to practice by working directly with patients, are now considering psychiatry as a career."[48] The administrator at Community Hospital reported that three out of ten interns one year were planning to go into psychiatry. One of the six American-trained interns in that year stated that he planned to become a psychiatrist. Another, who planned to take a residency in dermatology, had elected to spend one month in the adult outpatient psychiatric clinic at Community Hospital. He wrote a report of his outpatient experience claiming valuable experiences he gained there relevant to medical practice.

In response to one question, each of the Community Hospital house-staff members indicated that the intern should "instruct a patient about necessary medications." Three of them thought only the intern should do it. In a contrast, at University Hospital, half of the house-staff members indicated that "instructing the patient" was a task rightfully performed by at least three people in the hospital hierarchy, and one respondent wrote along the margin of the questionnaire: "our social service handles all these problems."

High standards for "adequate performance," priority for awareness of what is not known, and recognition of the intricacies of some social and psychological aspects of patient care, specialization and, colleague orientation may all tend to make the intern at University Hospital less comfortable than the Community Hospital intern about taking on full responsibility for some aspects of care.

An attending physician in an out-of-state university hospital discussed his hospital's difficulty in introducing interns to psychiatric consultations for patients. He said the problem was, "first, to introduce them to the idea of consultations; second, to wean them away from using them as a substitute for responsibility." The highly specialized team of medical and paramedical people available to contribute their special skills may at times be allowed to stand between the intern and his patient—especially when the intern approaches an area where he feels unsure of himself. Possibly, also, some details of patient's comfort, physical or emotional, at times slip through the network of various people responsible for him in the teaching hospital.

A former Community Hospital intern described the difference she noted between Community Hospital and a large university-affiliated hospital where she had been a clinical clerk. "In a place like that [University Hospital] you would have a whole hierarchy taking care of the patient. There were social workers, physiotherapists, occupational therapists . . . so you *could* assume that someone else would take care of paying attention to the patient's feelings."

Striving to make scientific advances on the one hand, or on the other, devoting one's professional life primarily to the care of "average" patients, can give rise to real differences in perspectives. Some physicians at Community Hospital feel their way is preferable, that emphasis on specialization necessarily implies a narrowing of interest in the patient. However, it is not simply a matter of selective recruitment of a personality type that goes into specialization. It is also *not* that the training makes the man narrow. Rather, as we have seen, the social context makes for specialized focus and facilitates consultation. As Robert Ebert noted, "I have never been convinced that the physician concerned with the science of medicine was any less concerned for his patient than his less scientifically oriented counterpart of a generation ago . . . There are probably as many 'kindly old specialists' as there are 'kindly old family physicians.'"[49] But the social context can increase the chances that the physician will *seem* to the patient to be oriented to narrow or wide interests. It may be that what some laymen's stereotypes refer to is simply difference in style. At times it may even be that a concerned manner is a cloak that makes the charlatan look like a dedicated physician to some patients.

Gateways to the Hospital Where Norms Conflict

Emergency room duty in the two hospitals offers an example of patterned differences in response to the same assignment in the two environments. Work in the emergency room of a hospital, and service as admitting officer, perhaps put the intern or resident in closer touch with the lay community than most of his other assignments, with the possible exception of the outpatient clinic. In a sense, the emergency room is used by some as they may have previously used a family doctor.[50] Mothers call from their homes for help or advice; press or police may become involved with tragic or unusual events. The person arriving for help is not as yet as separate from the community of the well and active as he is when he has a hospital gown, bed, diet, bed pans, and charts, and when his employer, family, and friends know him as "sick and hospitalized."[51]

Everywhere, the emergency room and to some extent also the outpatient department stand as gateways to hospital admissions. In any hospital where the intern or resident serves as admitting officer on emergency room duty, there is the possibility of selective admissions. Even in a municipal hospital, the resident decides whether the patient is sick enough for hospitalization. In the private hospital, ability to pay may influence admission. Also, chronic patients may be referred to veterans' hospitals or to other federal, state, or county hospitals.

Pride in performing well as an admitting officer seems to rest on quite different criteria in the two hospitals. In the University Hospital it derives more from demonstrated ability to screen patients effectively; in Community Hospital it relates more to being able to *accept* all patients who need to be in the hospital. It should be clear that selective screening is by no means the norm among affiliated hospitals and open admission is not the invariable rule among nonaffiliated hospitals. I use the fact of screening at University Hospital not because it is so common, but because where it does exist, it seems of some consequence.

The Community Hospital's administrator explained that admission was based pretty much on need of the patient to be hospitalized at this hospital, though they "try not to take on cases" that were obviously chronic problems, referring them to nearby state hospitals for chronic care. A resident at Community Hospital said any patient coming in with a note from an attending physician "would of course be admitted." An intern at another community hospital expressed what seemed to be the attitude of the house staff toward this admission policy: he said, proudly, that as far as he knew, "Not a single patient needing hospitalization had been refused admission during the previous year."

Moreover, physicians in Community Hospital expressed preference for their admission policy as best serving the teaching needs of interns and residents. The chief of one service said he thought interns should work "with all patients who arrive for admission rather than with those selected and worked over." Community Hospital interns and residents, more often than University Hospital house-staff members, said they thought physicians at their stage of training *should* see a "representative sample" of patients rather than those screened for teaching purposes.

The resident at University Hospital believes that all people who are ill and come to him for help should be cared for. But he has other hospitals to refer them to, and the resident's colleagues at University Hospital, whose esteem he desires, can exert daily pressure and potential future sanctions that may hold him to the conviction that screening patients is the "right thing" for him to do.

One resident at University Hospital spelled out his practical need of approval from the house-staff members he would be seeing daily, and indicated the priority he tended to use when exposed to contradictory demands. He was serving as admitting officer, and experiencing some of the cross pressures—from families and patients wanting to be admitted and from house-staff members demanding that patients be screened. The University Hospital resident said, "You are caught between many people. First, you are under pressure from the persons with whom you will have to have good relations all year [the peer group]; then you are caught between them and the patients who want to be admitted and who feel a great deal [is] at stake; then you are caught between the doctors who call and say they have to have a patient admitted right away." The resident then said he would be more influenced by an attending physician who was from "inside" the hospital rather than one from "outside." But he reemphasized the significance of approval from house-staff members of his specialty—whom he would be seeing daily—as he made difficult decisions about admitting patients. Later in the day, as he went about his duties as admitting officer for his service, he did refuse a patient for whom an attending physician had requested admission.

The University Hospital resident has only three weeks of emergency-room duty. Some comments suggest this three-week tour is likely to involve considerable strain on him. "It couldn't be longer," or "they would become paranoid." Some people in the hospital said they consider even two weeks almost the limit of time the resident can work there without making some adjustment in his commitment to screen patients—or some alteration in responsiveness to his patient's needs. Residents described their feelings of distress over having to disappoint sick patients. One, who served early in the year as admitting officer, ran into his chief resident who asked how he was getting along. The admitting officer smiled ruefully and said, "Where do you go to resign?" Residents who were steadfast in supporting the teaching goals as they served in the emergency room received support: "He is steady." "He is a pretty dependable fellow." One resident reported he could tell whether the admitting officer currently on duty was "doing a good job" by walking on the floors in his service and seeing what kinds of patients were there.

If residents on admitting duty "get too soft" and admit "routine cases" they bear the brunt of jokes and negative comments from their house-staff group. The admitting officer's daily rounds of each ward, to assess the number of beds available, give his house-staff group ample opportunity to let him know immediately whether or not they approve his admissions from the preceding day. These daily and vocal reminders of teaching commitments can bolster the resident's resolve when he might otherwise tend to adjust to pressures, from outside, and from his inner desire to respond to patient's hopes and needs or to insistent pleas from a family. Priorities at University Hospital may at times press the resident to resist some expectations of laymen. The priorities of Community Hospital more closely parallel those of the laymen.

The intern at Community Hospital serves a month in the emergency room, and he works there throughout the year on some of his nights on duty. Unlike University Hospital, Community Hospital does not regularly expose residents to the stressful experiences of trying to satisfy two conflicting expectations in the emergency room. Opportunity to work there is highly appreciated.

The administrator at Community Hospital spoke of "allowing" the intern these extra experiences on emergency-room duty throughout the year, and interns seem to share his high evaluation of this experience. One intern said he was very glad he had a chance to go back to emergency-room duty later in the year, after he had gained more confidence. A general practitioner, who had been an intern at Community Hospital, heard the intern's comment and said, "You're right, you'll be very glad you had that experience."

The community expects the hospital to admit anyone who is sick, and interns at Community Hospital use this expectation as their basic criterion for admitting patients. When he serves in this mediating position between hospital and community, the intern receives approval for conformity to some lay expectations. Moreover, the Community Hospital intern who plans to be in practice by himself soon is likely to be particularly eager for emergency-room duty. He may feel a more urgent need to learn to face emergencies alone than his colleague at University Hospital who plans several more years of training. Comments of house-staff members in both hospitals suggest they are aware of the potential significance of work in the emergency room. At University Hospital, the house-staff members seem less urgently to need to take on responsibility single handed, although they recognize it as valuable. They are more occupied with learning medicine. They have several more years, or a lifetime, of work with colleagues. In contrast, the intern at Community Hospital seems more confident that he knows enough. His concern is for chances to learn how to apply it. Emergency room duty thus has a very different position in the two hospitals. At Community Hospital it has top priority, and at University Hospital it holds a more marginal position.

Orientation meetings at Community Hospital provide much information about work in the emergency room which may stimulate the intern's interest in that duty, and at the same time provide him with practical directions. During orientation meetings, one physician described the relatively high incidence of admission of small children who have consumed cologne or miscellaneous pills around Christmas because visiting grandmothers have gotten out of the habit of protecting offspring against curiosity and oral inclinations.

Community Hospital's Poison Control Center also provides the intern with means of offering help in a hurry for many problems that will be brought to him. At one orientation meeting, the hospital anesthetist described the center. "The Information Center has made quite a little impact on the community . . . You can cope with most problems which will be presented to you in emergency."

Contributing to the positive evaluations of emergency room experience at Community Hospital are the individual arrangements developed around that service, and supported by authorities in the hospital. The value climate and social structure of Community Hospital, and the hospital's close ties with the local community contributed to making it possible for Community Hospital to develop one of the first poison control centers in the country. Three of the "old timers" in the hospital who were often cited by house-staff members as individuals who demonstrate initiative and willingness in helping the intern with specific problems—the anesthetist, the biochemist, and the pharmacist—created the poison control center where laymen and physicians can call for consultation or treatment. Those same three individuals also let the intern know they are available in an emergency. The development of this center may exemplify the type of innovation to be expected where there is emphasis on the individual initiative and arrangements found at Community Hospital.[52]

Differences in reaction to emergency work between the two hospitals is obviously related to the difference in plans that house-staff members have for their next few years. Less obvious, but possibly just as important in explaining the marked divergence in reaction to such work is the different priorities given to medical norms in the two hospitals. When the intern or resident at University Hospital is exposed to the full force of lay expectations, he may be made uncomfortably aware of the conflict between medical norms. We have discussed the many ways that the norm of the open mind, emphasis on relay learning, and graduated specialization are protected and reinforced on the specialty wards of University Hospital. These priorities that some University Hospital members have come to accept may be challenged with special force in the emergency room. But the Community Hospital physician, whose environment has provided encouragement and many reminders to reinforce priority of the "total patient," and many experiences in working as a physician alone, is in a sense better armed to meet some expectations of the layman.

VIII | Patient and Physician

Three fourths of the Community Hospital respondents, but *none* of the University Hospital respondents said they attached "great importance" to "ability to establish rapport with patients." This is consistent with a tendency for house-staff members at University Hospital to speak of "our patient," in contrast with the clarity with which nurses and interns at Community Hospital refer to "Dr. Jones's patient."

We have discussed the paradox that the friendly atmosphere of Community Hospital does not necessarily indicate a high incidence of friendship formation within house-staff group. Tending to compete with his fellow house-staff physicians for attention, the intern in the "friendly environment" must learn to get along with the patients as well as the nurses, attending physicians, and others throughout the hospital. The relevance of his relationships with these people is possibly greater when the intern lacks close ties within the house-staff contingent.

The number of initial histories and physicals the Community Hospital intern takes from private patients and his experience on emergency room service provide opportunities to practice getting along with a variety of patients alone and on first encounter. Chances are relatively good that such an intern will be somewhat alert to patient evaluations of his performance.

Both opportunity and pressure to take note of patient evaluations may help the Community Hospital intern to move with minimum problems of adjustment toward private practice, in which he must have some patient approval for success. To the extent that he does look to private practice in the very near future, he seems particularly susceptible to the judgments of his patients. He cares about learning to "get along" easily with patients, even the "hostile" ones.[1] Working more often alone, and with more articulate patients who at times are effectively demanding, the intern prepares for the physician's role as the community defines it. In contrast, at University Hospital the intern tends to have more occasion to lead his ward patients to adopt a role that the house staff defines.

Commitment to "rapport" and the patient-physician relationship introduces a special problem that may be generated when physicians become very concerned with approval from patients. The admirable practice of medicine by individual physicians, somewhat apart and insulated from visibility by other doctors, may demand that the physician become particularly responsive to "his patient." Norms of the medical Code of Ethics reinforce the commitment of doctor to his patient.[2] Patients who speak of "my doctor" as though he were irreplaceable, and some who brighten perceptibly when their doctor arrives, provide the reward of adulation the physician may be loath to jeopardize. With rather high "psychic income" from establishing rapport and "caring for" the patient in a double sense, the practitioner may become so committed to the relationship that he is over zealous in maintaining it.[3]

If the physician-patient relationship is very important to him, the physician may be willing to extend himself heroically, whether or not any of his colleagues can observe him. But such a physician can at times resemble a jealous mother who reacts with anger when a third party of any sort seems to threaten the relationship with her son. Dr. Holmes observed, "Doctors are the best-natured people in the world, except when they get fighting each other."[4] Some of the affect generated in arguments over the "patient-physician relationship," and over an individual patient who is considered "stolen" by a colleague, may be more fully understood as partly emerging from threats to self-esteem. Disagreements over "my patient" at times refer to nonpaying patients, and the arguments over the right of the physician to have the decisive word in treating the patient suggest that the more readily visible reward, money, is not always the key factor. A professor at one medical-school evaluated the bases for disagreements between local practitioners and the full-time professors at his hospital: "Basically, I would say that ego and economics create the kind of antagonism we have here. It isn't just that these people really lose patients, or feel any kind of pressure, as much as it is that they *fear* that they will lose patients; and also, they are embarrassed when they have to tell a patient that they can't admit him [to the medical-school hospital]." Another full-time professor reported: "The local practitioners in the community, I think, built up a tremendous defense for their own prestige with their individual patients."[5]

Patients may not be referred to a specialist when they should be; patients may be admitted to a hospital where the physician has admitting privileges, rather than where their problem might best be handled. Thus commitment to the relationship may help the doctor's responsiveness to his patient, but as with other commitments, the relationship can become an end in itself.[6] When this happens, some larger medical goals get temporarily lost.

Styles of Communication

In medicine, as elsewhere, breadth of responsibility, compassion, and concern is separable from a concerned *manner* and an air of sympathy. Nothing assures that the compassionate physician will not cause necessary—and sometimes unnecessary—pain or disquietude. He might, therefore, seem to patients to be callous or unsympathetic. On the other hand, a polished manner, an air of assurance and competence and sympathetic gestures and sounds can be an acquired manner that may or may not reflect concern. Clute observed: "One doctor was proud of his ability to appear relaxed before patients and said that he acted as though he had 'all the time in the world' with the result, he said, that very few of them noticed that he spent only about two minutes with them on the average.[7] The disapproval implied when some physicians refer to a staff member they think has "a bedside manner" points to the difference between having a quality and the *appearance* of having the quality. It is even possible, as Erving Goffman points out, that one can become so preoccupied with presenting the appearance of skill, the show of competence, the appearance of concern, that actual performance suffers.[8]

Teaching rounds in large affiliated hospitals are frequently cited as a source of potential stress for patients.[9] Rounds should also be considered from the perspective of the manner and style of dealing with patients they facilitate and present for emulation. As Milton Davis suggests, "One of the tasks that faculty often neglect is teaching students how to behave with patients. The data . . . suggest one reason for this neglect, that is, that the faculty could benefit from similar instruction."[10] As an example of needed teaching, the story is told about Robert Loeb's housestaff rounds at Bellevue. A resident asked whether it was to determine the temperature, moisture, or strength of the arm that Dr. Loeb shook hands with a patient on rounds. The physician's response was. "Gentlemen, the thing that I am doing is greeting another human being."[11]

Too often, however, the price of taking the time to reassure a patient on rounds is an opportunity lost for the intern to hear something important that the professor is saying about the physical complications of the same patient. At one bedside, a teaching group of seven people stood talking over a patient. Two members disconnected the tube leading to the patient's respirator so they could take a reading. No one explained the process to the patient. Obviously frightened, the patient strained to see what was being done with the respirator behind him. The group, intent on discussion of this patient's physical problem, moved to the next patient, leaving the nurse to reconnect the respirator.

The new intern whose patient this was, stayed for a moment, put his hand on the patient's arm, saying, "You are doing fine, Mr. Smith, I'll be back after rounds to talk with you." Because this intern took seconds out to reassure his patient, the man in distress, he missed what was being said about the medical aspects of his assigned case. This was early in the intern year for the young man whose medical school had devoted hours of curriculum time, efforts of professors and planning committees toward intelligent and sometimes creative efforts to sharpen awareness of the social and emotional aspects of illness. Thus, training and inclinations encourage attention to the patient's need for reassurance or explanation. However, in this case, when the intern responded appropriately he was not rewarded, for he didn't hear what the professor said. At other times in this setting, the intern may find repeatedly that he has missed out on something he values because he was responding to a patient's emotional reaction, or observing social amenities.

The social context creates occasions for rewards and losses that support certain aspects of medical manners and behavior over some other aspects. It is *not* that excellence of medical standards or specialization in a teaching hospital blunts compassion in a dedicated physician. It is, rather, that the physician already tending to handle the patient's fears by denying them, may be assisted in the unfortunate direction by environmental factors that facilitate his moving away via respectable concentration on discussion of the disease.

In all hospitals interns and residents sometimes emulate the style of an attending physician they respect. In one community hospital, an attending physician walked away from a bedside without a parting word, leaving the patient sitting up in bed. His three house-staff members followed him. None paused to say anything to the patient or to ask whether he wanted to have his bed adjusted to where it had been when they arrived.

As these two situations illustrate, some defect in manners can occur in hospitals, large and small, affiliated and nonaffiliated. However, the incidence may be less in environments where many private patients are seen by many attending physicians in private practice. As Eliot Freidson suggested, the organization of medical practice influences the way in which doctors perform their role. He found that doctors in solo practice are more likely to emphasize that part of their role which caters to the patient's need for "personal interest," while doctors in group practice tend to emphasize medical competence in diagnosis.[12]

As we saw in Chapter VII, the more articulate and secure patients sometimes do "call" a doctor up short if they feel he lacks tact or is impolite. Working a good deal with private patients gives the intern more experience to try his "social" skills, and Community Hospital offers the physician-in-training more reminders to be pleasant to the person who is a patient and more experience with meeting patients, particularly private patients. With this experience and the many role models at Community Hospital who are in private practice, chances are good that the intern there will become skillful at getting along with patients on brief encounter.

An aspect of "successful performance" for the physician with a private practice at Community Hospital may be to appear busy without seeming to be unduly rushed with any one patient—to be "friendly" and "nice." Probably few patients or their families like to feel their doctor is rushing to get away from them—any more than they like to think of him as having no other patients who want to see him.

In our nationwide survey, more house-staff members in the small nonaffiliated hospitals than in the large affiliated hospitals said they almost never encountered a hostile patient. This may be due to the difference in the distribution of the patients on hospital wards who often object to being used as objects for teaching and research. It is likely, however, that in part this reflects the intern's perception and his facility in handling patients. These are also the interns who meet many patients from various ranks briefly and without another physician present, and the ones who seem most likely to say "most any patient is interesting."

This does not mean that house-staff members at University Hospital are not concerned about patient feelings, as the following excerpt from my field notes shows:

Two interns and a resident, on their regular morning rounds, stopped by the bedside of one very old man. He said he was feeling better and they all congratulated him. He coughed and the resident put his hand gently on the patient's shoulder and said: "J., remember what to do when you cough? Cover your mouth. That's better." The patient's intern pointed to an oxygen cone and asked if the man remembered how to use it when he had a coughing attack. The patient said he did, but the intern showed him again to be sure, and the old man followed the intern with almost adoring eyes. As the house-staff members were leaving this patient's bedside, the resident patted the man's hand

and said, "J., you are our therapeutic triumph." The old man looked pleased but said: "I don't know what that means." The resident explained, "It means that we are proud of you and the way you are doing. You are a good patient."

Many interns and residents on this service at University Hospital seemed to have developed considerable skill in handling ward patients. They often made sure through repeated efforts that patients would understand simple things they needed to know for cooperation in their treatment. These house-staff members often reassured patients and protected them from uncertainties and potential anxieties, in ways similar to the manner of their chief of service as he approached patients in staff conferences.

In both hospitals, individual house-staff members did at times demonstrate tact and ability to handle emotional distress. The difference in the patterns of the two hospitals lies in the range of facility to manage all kinds of patients with seeming assurance and ease.

Another aspect of the physician's manner in dealing with patients is his presentation of himself as someone who is a technically competent authority. Here, too, it is possible that a clinician can learn to be effective in conveying the appearance of knowledge and competency, an appearance that far exceeds the reality. Community Hospital interns may come rather quickly to feel they need to present the patient with signs of their own skill and authority, and to convey attributes that patients often use in evaluating a physician's performance.[13] When intern and patient meet in more ambiguous authority relationships, the intern may be especially concerned about setting the scene for exchange to show that he can be effective, that he knows what he is doing. The Community Hospital administrator reported that one intern had complained early in his year that he "did not receive enough deference" in the hospital. Such complaints, and the communication patterns following them, may occur less often where rank and authority differences are relatively clear. Where the stage is set in advance, as it often is on University Hospital wards, the house-staff member has fewer occasions where he may feel a need to establish his authority vis-à-vis the patient. In the large teaching center, relatively low-status patients are often seen by physicians who can be sure of comparatively high position both in the hospital and in the medical community, and who at times approach patients with the reinforcement of a house-staff group. One physician, in discussing the potential advantages for interns' experiences with private patients, claimed that the private service provided a greater trial of the individual's social adaptability than did ward services.[14] Also, the house-staff member's relatively low economic position vis-à-vis the private patient is probably more often a matter of relevance in the smaller setting of Community Hospital.[15]

Compliance with Medical Orders

The need for layman and physician to share some ideas about their mutual obligations and rights is obvious. When they don't, the physician's best efforts can be frustrated, and the patient can be disaffected and discouraged so that he is not helped as much as he otherwise could be.

The many studies on compliance with medical orders and on drop-outs from outpatient clinics should be taken seriously, for they reveal some major gaps between physician and patient when they meet presumably to work together to determine the best solution to a medical problem.[16] The two learning environments of this study seem to provide differently for the development of the physician's awareness of the need to consider noncompliance as a potentially significant element in diagnosis and care. Beyond that, the intern and resident's work in two environments provides different chances that medical recruits will become skillful at inducing necessary compliance with the ambulatory patient.

The layman musters his courage to take himself or a family member to a clinic. Sometimes he waits a considerable time in an unattractive, crowded place to see a doctor. He may be called by number when his "turn" finally comes. But frequently something happens that leads him not to return for the next appointment. Psychiatric clinics have special problems, and they may give the person interested in patient-physician relationships strategic entry for study. With psychiatric patients, the relationship often becomes "the medicine" (sometimes the sole therapeutic instrument).[17] The quality of the relationship can be the vehicle for a return toward health, or the doctor's interaction with the patient may only reconfirm a patient's gloomy perception that there is no hope and "no reason" to follow the doctor's orders.[18]

Diabetes—a disease most often mentioned in discussions of compliance with medical orders—provides a special case for studying noncompliance because failure can have an immediate and visible effect. Also, there are objective measures available for control of the disease; medications and diet-control are largely up to patient and/or family away from the hospital. Moreover, the disease provides for possibilities of long-standing doctor-patient relationships. One physician said, "The control of the diabetic youngster is to a large measure evidence of the success of the physician . It is not always easy for the physician to face the fact that this control is not going perfectly well."[19]

The patient, not clearly understanding what he can expect in the stressful and ambiguous situation of illness, may search for symbols of the doctor's care and competence. Not perceiving them, he may withdraw from the situation—at times to consult someone who is less competent medically but more convincing. Vague fears of being rejected by the physician can also compound communication problems. Given the anxieties of illness and the chances for distortion, the scene is set for misperceptions, selective attention, and faulty memory for instructions. There is also the possibility for inappropriate ways of handling anxieties. Correlatively, there is great need for the physician to be aware of how the patient perceives what is going on, what the patient expects and what he hears.[20] As Minna Field observed a decade ago: "Under these circumstances, how patient could this man be in following out the medical recommendation for prolonged treatment and subsequent rest? Would his faith in medical treatment continue, or would he, under the pressure of economic conditions and worry about his family, return to work sooner than advisable only to face another exacerbation of his illness and yet another hospitalization?"[21] For some people the spiritualist, the druggist, the chiropractor, Christian Science and Jehovah Witness groups may seem more receptive, less threatening, and more immediate and comprehensible as a source of help.[22] For others, graphic television commercials will be taken as the preferred source of advice. Still others may follow a friend or relative's suggested remedy rather than taking prescribed medication. At least the friend listens to them and seems to understand.

Very often, the physician is unaware of just how ignorant he is of the patient's definition of the situation. Not knowing how the patient sees or comprehends advice and directions, not alert to how much the patient is denying, chances are slim that the physician will take the steps necessary to fill in information and correct misperceptions.[23] Nor will the physician's threats of dire outcome produce desired conformity when the patient's rational resources have already been put to rout by massive denial of his illness.

The portion of patients who fail to follow medical orders ranges from 15 to 93 percent, depending on the study. There is indication that doctors think more patients are taking medication as directed than actually is the case. For example, a study of tubercular patients on medication found that 96 percent of the patients indicated they were faithfully taking their prescribed medication. Their physicians judged that only about 80 percent of them were taking medication as prescribed. However, analysis of PAS and metabolites of INH indicated that only 72 percent had taken the drugs as prescribed on the day of their visit to the clinic.[24]

Another check on the relationship between a physician's estimate of his patients' behavior and an objective measure of behavior reports: "Twenty-seven ward residents estimated their individual patients' adherence to an antacide regimen (ATR). The physicians' estimates were then compared with counts of the bottles of antacid actually consumed by patients. The median patient took 46% of the prescribed medicine but the median physician's error of estimate was 32% . . . 22 overestimated their patients' ATR. Further, physicians were unable to distinguish those patients who adhered well from those who adhered poorly, even when the judgments were restricted only to those in which the physician indicated most confidence." The authors of that study conclude "The physician bases critical decisions in management and diagnosis on the patient's response to a therapeutic regimen. If he observed no response to a usually effective regimen, he may decide to change the treatment or he may even question his diagnosis. Yet, one reason a program may appear to be ineffective is that the patient is not following it."[25]

Milton Davis, who has provided a series of most interesting studies of noncompliance, reports, "Fifty-five per cent of the patient group expressed compliant attitudes and actually did comply; 22 per cent intended to, but did not comply; . . . 8 per cent actually followed their doctor's advice when they said they did not intend to do so; 15 per cent had no intention of complying and, in fact, did not." "Those with the greatest disabilities were found to be least willing and least likely to follow their doctors' orders." Davis raises the possibility that the nature of the patient-doctor relationship and patient attitudes predicts compliance better than such patient characteristics as education or religion.[26]

It looks as though the doctor can no more assume that the patient will comply with medical directives than the patient can assume assurance, explanations, comfort, and cure. In a study that evaluated physicians' actual performances it was found that the "student or faculty physician who receives lower performance ratings tends to see problems of the doctor-patient relationship in terms of the attributes and limitations of the patient."[27]

There are many areas of misunderstanding between patient and doctor, some needlessly large. "Because the purpose of tests is not explained to them, patients often begin to doubt that blood has to be taken for medical reasons. They think [and pass the word] that it is being taken only for purposes of training."[28] One Puerto Rican patient explained why she did not like to go to the public hospital: "If they take out a few drops of blood, you have to pay them although it's your own blood."[29]

As one patient in an affiliated hospital in Israel said, "The doctors here go their way and I go my way. They don't listen to me, so I don't listen to them. Dr. . . . [in another town] is my doctor and I am taking all his medicine even here in the hospital."[30] Results of this approach can be tragic. Robert Straus describes one case: "A middle-aged man was seen in a tumor clinic with an advanced carcinoma of the rectum. This patient had been seen in the same clinic two and a half years earlier and had been advised to undergo surgery for what was then diagnosed as a small polyp."[31]

The University Hospital puts the house-staff members less frequently in positions where they may be impelled to be aware of problems of noncompliance. Attending mostly to inpatients whose medication behavior is constrained by hospital routine, the house staff at University Hospital has relatively less experience that will effectively alert them to the need to attend to the patient's home situation as it may influence compliance. House-staff members whose most valued experience is with selected inpatients on a ward may be less often reminded of the need to be skillful in establishing the physician's authority and the legitimacy of expectations for compliance.

In contrast to an apparent tendency to devalue outpatient work at University Hospital, the practice-oriented Community Hospital staff appeared to prize the experience. An intern at Community Hospital volunteered, "When possible, I think all of us try to get to those [pediatric out-patient clinics]. For the most part you see the sort of thing you will see in practice and it is invaluable experience."

When the hospital relegates work with the ambulatory patient to lower prestige, it presents its house staff with a somewhat biased picture of medical practice. What is more, it reduces chances that trainees will make full use of the very place that could provide first-hand experience and training in attention to the total patient and his context. Such house-staff members can do well and learn much, but still know little about how to induce patients to both understand and accept medical advice and direction.

As Hans Popper observed, "With the changing role of the hospital, the out-patient department may be a more important teaching site than the wards." Yet at University Hospital, as in many other centers, the outpatient clinics are not particularly favored. As the Millis Report states, "The low status accorded the outpatient clinic naturally leads the student to the belief that ambulatory medicine is relatively unimportant . . . Merely adding a service of comprehensive medicine will not be enough, for everyone else would then relax and there would be little if any improvement of the present outpatient clinics."[32]

A tendency to downgrade work in the outpatient services of the teaching hospital is reflected in the system of appointments in some hospitals—different for outpatient and inpatient. An outside physician may have an associate-attending appointment to the outpatient department, but his rank in the inpatient service, if he has an appointment, is lower—as assistant attending. The most prestigeful senior physicians of the hospital, sometimes the best teachers and people house-staff members most admire, will seldom be found in outpatient work in some hospitals, although this is changing.

Pulling Together or Pulling Apart

People in University Hospital and other centers of medical education are concerned on behalf of "total patient care," "comprehensive care," and "continuity of care." There are many formal programs that emphasize these.[33] In the specialized practice of medicine, the segments of care that are separated out in science must in some way be brought back together, and they are sometimes rewoven most effectively.

Comments about overspecialization provide material from mass magazines from *Life* to *Look*. However, such negative comments are by no means new. Smollett complained in the eighteenth century that the patient was being "parceled out into small enclosures," a comment stimulated by the English legal distinction between the apothecary, the physician, and the surgeon. Even further back Herodotus wrote, "The practice of medicine is so divided among them, that each physician [in Egypt] is a healer of one disease and no more." One contemporary physician cites the advantages the contemporary patient has gained from much maligned division of labor in medicine, a division which is necessary for medical-scientific progress: "The typical oldtimer knew how and when to use his few drugs and how to apply sympathy, but beyond that he could do little. Over the course of a lifetime, a person is better off even in the hands of the iciest 'scientific monster' you can imagine than in those of the most compassionate oldtime doctor."[34]

In Chapter VII, I noted that there is a commonly held misconception that the medical scientist and the person whose work is highly specialized are necessarily unfeeling, and the general practitioner is necessarily compassionate. The belief should and does give rise to periodic disclaimers by medical educators. "No warm sympathetic person is frozen by research experience nor is a cold tactless individual thawed by general practice."[35] However, some attention should be given to social factors in hospital training experience which give credence to the stereotype. Different hospital contexts can produce many occasions that heighten awareness, or on the other side, that facilitate selective inattention to emotional and social factors relevant to patient care.

Two different attitudes of the physician can lead to a patient's justified perception that his doctor does not care enough about the social and emotional problems of the sick person. First, the physician can deny those aspects of patient's problems which he has been allowed to deny repeatedly throughout his training experience. A few lectures on the importance of social and emotional factors are a poor match to offset the sometimes urgent need for the doctor to deny problems that could threaten his self-confidence. This is doubly so when the internship and residency experience encourages the developing physician to prosper through show of brilliance on teaching rounds, and perhaps even to be rewarded most when he has spent time in the library and laboratory and least when he has spent time with his patient, or with a social worker trying to work out a problem for his patient. Second, the physician may be aware of social and emotional components of illness and recognize these factors as relevant to treatment success, but then be convinced that someone specializing in these areas, not himself, should assume responsibility for seeing that something is done. Once the appropriate experts are requested, physicians with this approach may back away from further attention to these elements.

The care and considerate attention that interns and residents at University Hospital often give their patients suggest that when its interns share their responsibilities with others, it does not stem from lack of concern. Such tendencies relate more clearly to commitment to specialization and the "team approach" as offering best care, and the fact that there are specialists available. Still, from the perspective of patients, what interns value as admirable acceptance of the limitations of individual skills may be viewed as "impersonality of specialists" or "narrowness," and the tendency for physicians to "parcel the patient out in segments."

Today's physician must consolidate and reconstruct from the patient's history, physical examination, and the reports that come through laboratory, social service, psychology, and other specialized sources. With reconstruction through consultation and joint efforts, the contemporary physician's potential for making intelligent decisions based on a wide range of data is improved. However, a new set of demands and problems is introduced. The internist, surgeon, psychiatrist, and other specialists have to learn not only to manage the patient but also the complexities of consultation and group efforts. In Chapter V we suggested that the social conditions that make for effective collaboration—frequent opportunities for informal consultation, chances for social approval for collaboration, abundant reminders of the unfortunate consequences of failure to consult, a value climate that holds relay learning in high esteem—all these are provided more abundantly at University Hospital than at Community Hospital.

The same social conditions may also give rise to occasions where some of the patient's needs may slip by unattended as each team member goes about his job. Without the team accompanying him, the physician in the smaller hospital can seldom assume "that social service takes care of all that." When a single doctor is alone with the patient, chances are better that the patient will volunteer information or questions, that the doctor will *hear* them, and that he will not assume that some specialist is handling the problems. On the other hand, the University Hospital context which encourages consultation and the team approach can support the physician's efforts at bringing many specialists to bear on his patient's problems.

An example from Lester Evans' discussion of crises in medical education, demonstrates what can happen to a patient whose physician retains a feeling of responsibility and at the same time is deeply commited to specialization and the team approach. "A 42-year-old husband and father, employed in heavy labor, suffers a cerebral vascular thrombosis that results in paralysis of his right side, and a speech impairment. He receives good emergency care during the acute comatose period immediately following the attack. Soon after he regains consciousness and stability, an active program of physiotherapy and speech therapy is instituted, first at his bedside and later in the appropriate clinic. Recognizing that the patient will be unable to return to heavy labor, his physician calls upon the rehabilitation center for assistance. While the patient is still hospitalized a rehabilitation team . . . social worker, psychologist, occupational therapist, physical therapist, work evaluation and vocational counselor [work] with him, his family, his physician and his nurses. Under the concentrated treatment [he learns to] walk with a leg brace and talk with only slight difficulty. After a vocational training course, sponsored by the department of vocational rehabilitation, he is placed in a full-time job as a timekeeper-clerk. Today he travels to and from his work unassisted and has resumed his role as a family breadwinner." Evans notes the converse of this: "the stroke victim who, lacking treatment and guidance to restore him to self-sufficiency, becomes an invalid, a ward of the state, and an agent of despair."[36]

Breadth of Responsibility and the Behavioral Sciences

We have observed how the University Hospital environment facilitates consultation between medical specialists. But we should consider use of psychiatric consultation as a separate phenomenon. At University Hospital and in some other centers, residents readily consulted and asked for help and advice from other specialists. At the same time, they seldom called for psychiatric consultation to help them solve problems and come to decisions about the best way for them to manage their own patients.

Studies that find a high incidence of somatic disorder in psychiatric patient populations, and also a high incidence of psychiatric disorder in populations of medical and surgical patients, speak eloquently for the need to incorporate psychiatric consultation as a viable part of training programs for the nonpsychiatrist.[37] Among the psychiatrists who have led efforts to bring psychiatric consultation and services into medicine, M. Ralph Kaufman points to the distance that psychiatry still has to go, although there are increasing numbers of psychiatric services within the general hospital. At the same time, studies of the use of psychiatric consultation and/or referral provide much evidence of confusion about—sometimes aversion to—the uses of psychiatry in medical practice.[38]

Four factors contribute to sometimes isolating the specialty of psychiatry from the rest of medicine. First, the intern and the resident in some hospitals may have had good experiences from consulting with hematologists, radiologists, and pathologists. But he may have had relatively little experience working closely with a psychiatrist on a patient's problem. Some hospitals that are superior in all other respects for house-staff training have no psychiatric service.[39] Psychiatry in some hospitals is a somewhat isolated department that does not supply consultation as speedily as it is provided by some other specialty sections. Occasional references to psychiatrists as "the nine-to-five doctors" refer to the relative tardiness of responses by psychiatrists to requests for consultation. Garber noted from his sample of physicians who were asked which sources gave them most knowledge of psychiatry that psychiatric consultations were a poor last; 83 percent of the general practitioners did not specify this source at all. Next to this least-mentioned source came medical schools.[40] It sometimes happens that interns are told by their peers and taught by experiences that a request for psychiatric consultation may mean little more than several days' delay of discharge while the patient waits to be seen by a psychiatrist.

The second factor that works to separate psychiatry from medicine is that other physicians may see psychiatrists as more atypical than they actually are.[41] Funkenstein characterized three types of students at Harvard Medical School: the scientist, the practitioner, and the psychologically minded. Psychiatry is the goal of the latter; half of them decided on psychiatry before entering college. Many of these had majored in the humanities and they have higher verbal aptitudes than the other students.[42]

Student images of specialties do change in some schools and often not to the advantage of psychiatry, which sometimes ends up with the lowest rating except for dermatology.[43] A research team at the University of Oklahoma reports, "It can be seen . . . that as medical knowledge and experience increase, the image of internal medicine becomes more positive whereas the opposite is true for the image of psychiatry."[44] Wives of medical students in one school follow the same pattern. Clinical students' wives rate each of six specialties lower than do the wives of preclinical students. But, the downgrading is "notably so for psychiatry, pediatrics, and obstetrics-gynecology."[45]

The psychiatrist with his halo slightly askew is not infrequently a subject of humor, and sometimes derision, within the medical profession, and this does influence students' attitudes toward psychiatry. When the intern never sees the internist consult a psychiatrist, or upon consultation he observes the internist doesn't listen or the psychiatrist doesn't appear till much later or doesn't help—that student is learning about psychiatry in medicine. But he is probably not learning what either the internists or the psychiatrists on the faculty hope for when they plan the curriculum and state school aims. Admonitions once a week are poor competition for a multitude of daily actions when the two sources convey competing messages.

Paul Kaufman describes some of the difficulties in making psychiatric consultation a meaningful part of the resident's work in a teaching hospital: "Frequently the phychiatrist must pass through a kind of test, to see if he is still really a doctor and thus a colleague; this involves more than simply demonstrating factual knowledge. The willingness to pitch in and assume responsibility is more important. However, demonstrating the possession of an adequate medical background and the ability to recognize gaps in one's current usable information is often a vital first hurdle to be passed in developing a useful relationship with the house staff."[46]

Another handicap in efforts to encourage meaningful use of psychiatric material and consultation is the content of the material, which may be threatening to students and to senior physicians alike. For this reason, the material presented by psychiatry is more subject to distortion by students.

Also, physicians as well as laymen may not consider emotional disturbances as illnesses that merit consultation. This is probably changing with the expansion of psychiatry in medical school curricula. Werkman notes that "a half century ago, psychiatry had an average of 30 to 40 hours in the entire medical curriculum; today most departments have 300 or more hours." The literature on the subject of how best to introduce medical students to effective use of psychiatry and principles of psychiatry is voluminous; but it often assumes that more is learned when more hours are devoted to the subject. There is still occasional evidence of something less than total success in efforts to integrate psychiatry and other behavioral sciences in medical education.[47]

Physicians' psychiatric consultations for their patients appear to fall into three types, resembling the responses to introducing psychiatric consultation that I observed among teachers in college preparatory schools.[48] First, there are physicians who may be specialists but who accept a wide range of responsibility for their patients, and who bring in a psychiatric consultant along with other consultants but without attempting to "dump" troublesome patients through consultation. The physician in charge of the stroke victim who was helped back to a productive life is an example of those physicians who fit the ideal or model of the "primary physician" described in the Millis Report.[49] Then there are physicians who are primarily oriented to their specialty and who see their responsibility to the patient as somewhat circumscribed—performance within the specialty. The resident who wrote, "Our social service takes care of all these things," expressed this orientation. With this conception of the physician's role, when a psychiatrist is called in, it may be primarily in order to have the patient transferred to the care of a psychiatrist.

Then there is the physician who may need to believe that he "knows human nature" and can therefore best handle his own patients—all except the "psychos" who—as a resident said in an interview—"are not reclaimable." The stereotype of the physician with this orientation is the "friendly old doctor." Though many of these physicians may handle psychiatric problems well and be of tremendous help to patients there is always the possibility of the physician going over his depth in this specialty area, as in any other. Milton Mazer found in the Island Community he studied that "approximately four times as many persons with significant psychiatric disorders remained in treatment with their general practitioners as were treated by a psychiatrist even though psychiatric outpatient care was readily and promptly available and geographically accessible, at low cost, to every inhabitant."[50] An intern in one community hospital expressed this orientation: "What I see and do not like is these people who see a problem outside their field and throw up their hands. This is not medicine. I guess the thing is to know when you really need consultation."

Community Hospital may help in the development of this third, friendly physician, type. University Hospital conditions facilitate the way of the specialist physician who may be more likely to refer *to* than to consult *with* psychiatrists. Other university-affiliated hospitals that have active liaison to bring senior as well as resident psychiatrists to each specialty may be in the best position to encourage house-staff patterns of close collaboration with psychiatrists.[51] For psychiatry to be maximally used toward total patient care, physicians in training need experience in frequent exchanges with psychiatrists who will consult regularly and not simply take the patient away or "get him out of the hair" of the other physician.

The Interesting Patient

Some comments from house-staff members both in Community Hospital and University Hospital suggest a tendency to see patients as "interesting" when they provide the intern or resident an opportunity to perform successfully within the value climate of his *particular* hospital. One study of a hospital found that patients whose behavior does not conform to the sick role as defined in that setting endanger the physician's self-concept and make him respond negatively.[52]

Howard Becker found that medical students tend to rank patients according to the extent to which the patient provides the novice physician a chance for success. "This perspective, which we believe to be an important one in medical culture generally, furnishes a basis for classifying and evaluating patients; those patients who can be cured are better than those who cannot. Furthermore, those patients who cannot be cured because they are not sick in the first place are worst of all."[53] A similar tendency occurred in another medical-school affiliated hospital: "patient's with 'uninteresting' [low-prestige] diseases were sometimes accused of belonging to a mental hospital rather than to this one. This indicates that psychiatry is sometimes assigned cases that seem unworthy of medical attention."[54]

In the University Hospital environment, where patients are "selected" and where learning and research are highly valued, an unusual finding provides the intern with an opportunity to display his medical knowledge of "latest findings," and at times the chance to perform as a teacher. The professor may invite him to present the case to medical students. An attending physician at University Hospital said about house-staff members: "What makes you a better doctor than the next is if you can pull a diagnosis that they miss . . . It is those few [patients] you concentrate on." An intern said: "The really interesting case is the one who is a *challenge* to diagnose." Other University Hospital staff members defined the interesting patient with attributes such as "unusual disease," "unusual manifestations of a common disease," "a good diagnostic problem." These patients at times offer potential for a research paper that can claim the attention of the medical-scientific community—or at the very least offer the intern or resident a chance to gain favorable attention on rounds. Thus, a patient may gain or lose the quality of being "an interesting" case. "You doctors! How your demeanor changes! There was a time when you all considered my case interesting, and you'd come to see me one after the other. Now I'm not an interesting case any more. So you all rush by like locomotives."[55]

At Community Hospital, house-staff members seem to evolve different definitions of the "interesting patient" as they progress through their internship. One intern was asked, late in her internship year what "interesting patient" meant. Her response was one of surprise: "This is a nonsensical question. Certain patient are interesting as people, certain as showing rare diseases, others as being a diagnostic problem, and others as being a therapeutic problem." Another responded: "A patient who has a unique problem from the medical point of view. However, the routine cases are interesting because of the psychological episodes precipitating the onset of the disease." One said: "A patient with whom a good doctor-patient relationship can be established and who can benefit in some way from such an arrangement." Nationwide, 70 percent of the house staff in large affiliated hospitals—but only a little over 50 percent of those in smaller community hospitals—said they would prefer a patient whose illness is entirely physical.

House-staff members in each hospital were aware that one could learn from work with any patient. In Community Hospital, however, there seemed relatively less emphasis on cases that might offer an opportunity to allow the intern or resident to display his knowledge, or to contribute something to the medical knowledge of his house-staff group or to scientific medicine in general. One intern at Community Hospital said: "Interesting patient . . . depends on what you discussed the previous week. You need these things refreshed in your memory in an organized fashion. Once in a while if they did get an exotic problem, it could be included."

The intern working with private patients sees relatively few cases that the University Hospital screening policy implicitly suggests are interesting. Interns and residents there occasionally express lack of enthusiasm for their experience on the private service, which they sometimes refer to as the "Gold Coast." Some of their tendency to downgrade work there may reside in the house staff's relative inability to get these patients to conform to the role as the house staff defines it. In addition, some of the attending physicians on private services seem to be more concerned with evaluations that laymen make than the University Hospital interns and residents feel is proper. This clash of definitions limits satisfaction with experience on private service. Beyond this, the intern has less "say" about treatment on the "Gold Coast." His authority is undermined by his relative youth, his financial situation, and the fact that he is not the patient's doctor. The term "Gold Coast" itself condenses the notion of a primitive situation where role partners are not adequately socialized, at the same time as it signals the wealth and potential power of many patients.

The chief resident on one service at University Hospital said: "Part of the 'rough time' for interns on the 'Gold Coast' derives from the fact that many of the patients think of the hospital as a hotel. They are frequently annoyed because they can't have steak when they demand it, or the hospital doesn't provide secretarial service when they want it . . . and often their attitude toward the intern is that he is a nuisance that they don't need to put up with." As one intern walked into one of the weekly staff conferences in this service, a fellow intern asked: "Where have you been working these days?" He answered, "Back in the Tower," referring to the private service. The first intern quipped: "You came back from a vacation just for *that*?"

These same interns and residents seem enthusiastic about their work on the wards where they have more time with each patient, more responsibility for diagnosis and treatment, where they can work as a team, *and* where patients may interfere less with their expectations. When house-staff members at University Hospital indicated their preferences for patients, over one third of them chose "down-and-out" patients. One of these respondents added a note after his selection of the "down-and-out" patient: "It helps me to listen!" The ward patients in this hospital do seem less likely than private "Gold Coast" patients to intrude their expectations effectively. Thus the intern is allowed to hold to behavior that reinforces the norm of "the open mind," ideals of "relay learning" and scientific discussion, *at the same time* that he is rewarded by patients' approval. Adjusted to the value climate of specialty work on wards at University Hospital, the house staff may experience the private service as a chilly and alien environment. This, in turn, has implications for future satisfaction of men trained at University Hospital.

Occasionally, a former University Hospital resident who returned either to visit or to see his private patient seemed to be almost apologetic about his present work. One reported to his friend, still a resident: "I'm just in practice." Another seemed defensive about the nonteaching hospital where he was an attending physician, "But there are sick people there, too."

Factors contributing to work that is rewarding for house-staff members on University Hospital wards can also create problems of discontinuity for those physicians who move toward private practice. The resident who follows house-staff training at University Hospital with a "successful" private specialty practice is likely to have to cope mostly with patients who would be admitted to the "Gold Coast." One attending physician from an out-of-state university hospital said: "The university hospitals do get selected and sifted patients, so the intern's concept of what the practice of medicine is really like will likely be disorted." Then he added that he felt this might make some physicians, trained in such an environment, unhappy in practice where they would be seeing primarily cases which by their former judgment would be considered uninteresting. Since few patients are disposed to see their own problems as uninteresting, communication problems between patient and physician may be aggravated if these physicians carry house-staff prejudices into their practice.

Crocks, Turkeys, and Gomers

At the other extreme from the interesting patient, the terms "crocks," "turkeys," and "gomers," are sometimes summary criticisms which express frustrations and stress that interns and residents experience in their particular setting.

House-staff members at University Hospital throughout the year tended to express annoyance over seeing "too many" patient who were "hypochondriac," "paranoid," with "psychogenic symptoms," and "the people who have nothing but psychogenic symptoms." These were the patients who seemed most likely to fall into the category of crock. One resident at University Hospital said: "I get exasperated when 90 percent [of the patients on one ward] are not reclaimable . . . social problems." At University Hospital the terms turkey and gomer, were heard less often than crock.

But in a county hospital with university affiliation, Hospital B, two separate interns, who said they knew the word crock from medical school, emphasized that they did not like it and did not use it. They said they did use turkey to represent the admitting officer's error in judgment because he had admitted someone who did not need hospitalization. On the first of July in this hospital a new intern said he didn't know the word turkey. A resident asked, "How about a gomer? They're the same." The intern nodded and said, "Oh, someone not as sick as the admitting officer thought at midnight." The summary criticisms turkey and gomer that were used at Hospital B carried very different meaning from the term, crock, as it seemed to be used at University Hospital.[56] Indeed, the county hospital with university affiliation admitted many patients who in a sense would have been dismissed with the label crock by at least a few staff members at University Hospital. But hospital charts of many alcoholics and the derelicts at Hospital B included multiple psychological and social components as part of the table of contents which was the guide to problems to be solved or clarified, or at least to be held in mind and acknowledged as yet to be solved.

Thus, in two university-affiliated hospitals, house-staff members expressed quite different approaches to patients with multiple psychological and social problems. Similarly among the nonaffiliated hospitals there is a wide range of house-staff attitudes toward such patients. In Hospital D, one intern said, "The interesting patient? That's a diagnostic problem, rare diseases, classical diseases, ones with dramatic results—like the lady with classical gout that cleared. Then we have the crocks and the turkeys. Crocks are patients who don't have anything wrong with them and who for various reasons . . . feign illness. Turkey is the same. A turkey admission is someone who shouldn't have come in—especially in the middle of the night. This is the time when most of the turkeys slip in. Mrs. F. qualifies as a first-class crock. She has got mental illness but she wants to be sick and she is a difficult problem because she takes her own medication . . . completely unrewarding because all they do is complain." But his fellow intern indicated that crocks might also have illnesses subject to treatment by the nonpsychiatrist. Asked what the word crock meant, he answered, "These people get sick and they usually get very sick because they have gotten the label of crock and nobody has taken their symptoms seriously enough. I followed a gentleman on psychiatry and he really looked sick, and it turned out he was." In another community hospital (Hospital C), an intern said, "By the way, crocks die of organic disease, too, and that is something to keep in mind."

In still another unaffiliated hospital, Hospital E, which I have described as having unusual success in recruiting interns and in keeping in touch with local practitioners, two interns sat over coffee chatting. Neither of them knew the terms turkey, or gomer, but they both knew the word crock. One said, "I like them. In fact, I got to be known as the crock doctor at . . . [the university hospital where he had worked as a fourth-year student]. If you can get through to them, you can do a lot for them. The one thing I found was that many of them turn out to have disease . . . just nobody had diagnosed it yet."

Several of these comments which suggest recognition that the "crock might be sick, too" are encouraging. These interns were aware, as one team of psychiatric consultants put it, "that positive findings, on either the physical examination, or the psychiatric examination, do not indicate that the patient must be categorized exclusively as either psychiatrically or medically ill."[57]

The Worlds of Town and Gown

University Hospital encourages a special kind of consulation, that is, within the teaching center and even within the nation-wide network of specialists in research, but not within its local community. Physicians at Community Hospital sometimes complain that when they refer to University Hospital or other teaching centers they are not being "listened to." No one cares what they know about the case, and they do not receive feedback when they refer "their" patients to the hospital.

In one out-of-state community, where a medical-school hospital had been recently introduced, local practitioners expressed resentment over their loss of prestige when the academics arrived in the community. A local practitioner in one community commented on the prestige ranking between those inside the university complex and the others who were outside of it. "Their wives always put this [university appointment] information into their obituaries, so I guess it must have some honorific value." Another described his unfortunate experience with people in his town's university hospital. "Let me tell you what happened to me once. I had a patient with serious kidney disease. I wanted the professor to see him. So, in preparation for that, I worked up a nice little history of the case. When I started to present this, the professor cut me short and said that wasn't necessary. He said he just wanted to see the patient. I had told him that the patient's kidney area was extremely tender. But he went in . . . probed . . . the patient cried. I was embarrassed by the whole episode . . . The point is that, had I been one of the clique, his attitude would have been different."[58]

One result of the difference in prestige of the two types of internships is that the physician from the smaller hospital may have some hesitancy about sharing his knowledge with colleagues from the teaching hospitals.[59] The difficulty is compounded when physicians with more prestige assume they can learn nothing of use from the local practitioner. (The patient may also be frustrated by having to recite his history repeatedly.) The physicians in the university hospitals thus lose a potential source of information about the history and life situation of the persons they are to examine. The physician from the outside is discouraged from trying to meet some of the university hospitals' standards as well as from trying to keep up-to-date through regular contact with the teaching and research center. A self-fulfilling prophecy can be set in motion by the tendency of some physicians of the university centers to denigrate the outsiders in local practice.[60] Not expecting much of good medicine, or much of value from them, the academic physician and his house-staff members are likely to behave in ways that do not enhance, but discourage, the best efforts of the local clinician.[61]

One professor in Patricia Kendall's study of eight "town-and-gown" communities reported:

"I don't belong to the county society, although I keep meaning to join. But I see how everyone in the community works at keeping the relationship [between educators and practitioners] good." This is the cosmopolitan physician we quoted before as saying, "I'm not sure about it, but I think so. I'm an outside here. I've been here for nine years."

Question: "You're an outsider after nine years?"

"Yes, in the sense that I'm not so concerned with the community as I am with national and even international developments. I'm not such a rah-rah man. I think in a way, this is good. It deprovincializes the departments."[62]

Where the relative prestige of training programs between affiliated and nonaffiliated hospitals interferes with productive communication between men in practice, interns and residents in both types may lose something. Young men from prestigeful training centers may miss a good potential source of information about daily practice. And interns, as well as attendings, in the community hospitals lose the benefits of pressures on behalf of standards and keeping up with medical advances being made in the large medical centers.

The introduction of a medical school in a community or a hospital can pose a double threat to local physicians. First, their own self-esteem may suffer from being in the relatively lower position of practitioner compared to professors. Second, the local physicians may experience an assault against their professional commitments to ethical practice. In one community different orientations and their related rewards contributed to a flare-up of conflict between town-and-gown physicians. One practitioner said, "We first had great difficulty with them [full-time professors] conforming to our local code of ethics about getting publicity. They did not seem to understand how we felt, and *we feel strongly about those things.*"

Patricia Kendall writes about this community: "A final important element in the practitioners' feeling that they are at a competitive disadvanage vis-à-vis full-time men is that, while medical ethics prohibit them from publicizing themselves and their activities, it is generally considered legitimate to publicize developments at the university—including its medical school. In some instances, this had led to violent disputes."[63]

There are contradictory expectations in the two worlds.

Within the ethics of colleagueship the influentials on the town side of medicine disapprove of publicity. Competition for patients is destructive of the colleague system. Within the ethics of science on the gown side of medicine, advances must be made the property of all and publicity is quite compatible within this ethic. Legitimate rewards for the creators in medical science include some form of publicity for a scientific advance or findings and such rewards help spur still more efforts toward scientific advance. However, the same rewards contribute less efficiently to some ends of daily medical practice.[64]

If more profitable exchange is to be possible between men from the two worlds, some understanding of differences in commitments—and the functions they serve for the two directions—is required. Some teaching centers offer and encourage local practitioners to come into the hospital for refresher courses, rounds, and lectures. The federal government is supporting programs for the general practitioner in special subjects. Some hospitals have started concerted efforts to reach practitioners in their areas, not only through courses but also by providing a program of active feedback when practitioners outside the hospital refer their patients to the hospital. But a few lectures, or taped and televised presentations have gross limitations compared with frequent exchange over cases that come within the purview of the two types of physicians.

An internist in one community discussed the problem: "I think the attitude on the part of the full-time attending staff at the hospital, that treating people who are sick is not somehow quite as fine as doing research or teaching—almost, in some cases, as though sick people are unclean—this gripes us who are in clinical medicine. You almost get the feeling sometime that those people who work on dogs and test tubes are somehow finer than the men who work on human beings . . . This whole problem boils down to C. P. Snow's two worlds—there are entirely different approaches to medicine. There are the men in teaching and there are the men of the world—the clinicians."

The comments of some local practitioners who had recently been made aware that the very basis of their own self-esteem—having many patients who valued them—"does not count" in the academic prestige system, resemble the pathos of a man who has discovered that neither he nor his work is what matters today. And some physicians who have abruptly been faced with the new medicine feel exactly this way. Clute reports his surprise that although so many general practitioners complained about long hours and lack of free time and although most were within a mile of another doctor "there was little evidence that they were attempting to improve the conditions of practice." "We were greatly disturbed by the attitude manifested by certain doctors that their patients *belonged* to them."[65] This commitment is not just a relic of the past. Results from a 1956 nationwide survey of over 1,000 medical students indicated that the principal satisfaction these students anticipated achieving through their medical careers related to doctor-patient relationships.[66]

Somewhere in the possible varieties of environments for training and for later practice there must be conditions which can foster development of more clinicians who will retain their concern for keeping up-to-date and for excellence in the science of medicine. For this, there must be discourse and opportunities for the clinician to feel at one with medical colleagues who concentrate on teaching and advancing science. Patients deserve to have someone in medicine who is willing to commit himself to comprehensive concern for the patient and who is at the same time competent and knowledgeable—not a denigrated stepchild of the educational enterprise.[67]

IX | The Uses of Diversity

Advances generate new demands and the medical system sometimes creaks and groans under the strain of accommodating to unfamiliar functions and to new occupations that emerge within and around it. Past training in specifics is made inadequate, and old habits and perspectives can incapacitate the professional asked to perform in a new context and with new partners.[1]

A stable base of professional identification and supple relationships within the profession are needed to support the vibrations and shifts of changing science, technology, and social roles and relationships. When the profession fails to bring its recruits to identify with it, some doctors drift off to the outskirts of the medical care system where they practice relatively beyond the influence of the medical academy and its hospitals. Without viable relationships between physicians who follow different careers in medicine, each segment narrows and chances for productive exchange diminish. Men deep inside the research and teaching centers may become far removed from some of the realities that their students will eventually have to face in practice, with the consequence that expectations and goals are set so high they discourage attempts to attain them. The hospital-educational system thus must provide some common experiences and possibilities for identification for physicians who will then pursue widely diversified careers.[2] But at the same time, each of the several different career directions that physicians are asked to follow will have to be sustained by its own specific ethos and provided its own manageable priorities between conflicting norms.

In the past, when a larger share of physicians were training for a lifetime of solo practice, either general or specialized, all hospital training programs could more reasonably follow similar lines. Then, many of the illustrious physicians who taught were volunteers, supported by their own successful practice. They were appropriate role models for the many interns and residents whose life work would be in private practice. Today, however, it seems increasingly apparent that a few different types of programs in appropriately different types of hospitals may be required to develop the best within each distinct career line, and provide the variety of medical services presently required.[3] Environments that enhance the development of the medical scientist may not be as felicitous for the maturation of the physician who plans to be a clinical specialist in private practice. The program and hospital environment that provide maximum teaching, support, and encouragement to develop physicians for community medicine may be still different. Yet another type of hospital learning environment may encourage the development and maturation of the family, or primary, physician.

As the medical system incorporates more distinctly different career orientations, the question, "Which single type of hospital, which type of house-staff training program should be the model for the country?," becomes less appropriate. The more appropriate question will seek to determine which type of hospital and which training program can best support the *particular* career direction—and still keep it related to the whole of medicine. Beyond this and related closely to it, the next question should search for types of hospital structures that can be utilized to continue a lifetime of support, education, and social control for excellence within each of the major career directions.

Separation of Function by School and Hospital

Changes in the population of students who enter medical school presage something of a new division of labor in the medical system. More students arrive at medical school with advanced training in biology and the physical sciences rather than with the more general "pre-med" concentration.[4] More medical students come to their house-staff training with more advanced and specialized training. The straight internship, which is a rather recent step toward early specialization, is being surpassed by changes within medical school to allow for still earlier differentiation. We have referred to the three types of medical students that Daniel Funkenstein describes in a Harvard sample: the student-scientist (and there is an increasing number of these), the student-clinician (losing numbers), and the student-psychiatrists. There is a fourth type emerging—the social-scientist physician. As Funkenstein observes, "Very few medical schools, if any, would have the necessary resources—not only in funds but in personnel—to develop all . . . areas of study. For this reason, it would be desirable for each medical school to decide whether it would educate only one type of physician or whether it would be able to offer training in 2 or even in all . . . areas. Once this decision was made, the school's admission policies could be adjusted so as to fit students with career plans appropriate to its particular curriculum."[5]

If the social structure and value climate of the medical school and hospital are as significantly different as they seem, there are reasons beyond the limited resources of funds and personnel that argue for specialization within the network of training institutions. The structure and climate best designed to foster attitudes, behavior, and identification with science and research is not necessarily the environment best equipped to develop family physicians who are sensitive to social and emotional factors in illness. Careful attention to the social structure and value climate of house-staff training programs could result in support for several different forms of hospital learning environments, each offering reinforcement for excellence within the particular medical careers fostered in that hospital.

Diverse hospitals with academic support for their special training and service functions might also provide more effectively for continuing education of the type of physician each specializes in training. They could develop channels for exchange between university and graduate physicians who follow the particular careers they have helped to develop. Permeable boundaries between the academic community and local practitioners may be more likely when there are respected teaching hospitals of more varied forms that can improve chances for match between more interns and their learning environments. It is not surprising, when hospital and intern have been mismatched, to learn that later ties between the physician and his training hospital are tenuous, if they exist at all.

Pellegrino states the present dilemma of medical education: "The plight of the medical educator is very much like that of the White Knight [in *Through the Looking Glass*] as he tries to equip his young crusaders for their service to society in the fight against physical ills. So many things are available which might be useful and so varied are the needs of an anxious society that, in desperation, he tries to provide for all eventualities. The one weapon missing is that of discrimination, a most difficult business since the nature and magnitude of all the future battles is largely unknown. Yet we must somehow avoid the current practice of encrusting our curricula with successive exposure to an increasing array of clinical specialties, subspecialties, techniques, and 'learning experience.' We need to teach the knight how to stay in the saddle and at least hold on to his lance."[6] The same may be said for the over-all planning of the house-staff period of training, and possibly a first step toward discrimination is to analyze the essentials of social reinforcements, as well as the substantive material that should go into the developing of physicians along different career lines.

Continuing Medical Education

The Millis Report states: "Medical practice has changed greatly. Yet the judgment is widely expressed, in and out of medicine, that the changes have not been profound enough to keep pace with the growth of medical knowledge and the rise in society's expectations and demands. The current problems of medicine are in large measure problems created by its own success . . . It is now widely agreed that for the physician to remain highly competent, his education must not terminate at the end of a formal residency, but must continue as long as he practices."[7]

It becomes less and less feasible for the medical educator to expect he can give the student, then the intern and resident, all the specifics the doctor will need in ten years. By the same token it becomes more urgent that the developing physician learn the habit of meaningful consultation and become committed to acquiring knowledge, regardless of the career direction he takes.

The physician-educator of fifty years ago could concentrate on content and be reasonably assured of two things. First, he would continue ahead of his students in the sciences he was teaching. Second, his experiences in treating patients through the years would be of interest to his students, most of whom hoped for a private practice. The man who teaches an advancing science today has a greater challenge. His students will go in several different career directions and he cannot cover all directions effectively. Moreover, he cannot rest with conveying facts and believe the student will have the information needed for a lifetime of practice. The new professor must encourage discontent with present knowledge but still provide the individual student with a foundation secure enough for effective action.

A hospital enviroment that consistently provides rewards for the inquiring attitude, thorough and detailed chartwork, and for teaching can serve well for the physician who moves toward teaching and research. Osler wrote, "The seclusion of the student life is not always good for a man, particularly for those of you who will afterwards engage in general practice, since you will miss the facility of intercourse upon which often the doctor's success depends. On the other hand, sequestration is essential for those of you with high ambitions proportionate to your capacity. It was for such that St. Chrysostom gave his famous counsel, 'Depart from the highways and transplant thyself into some enclosed ground, for it is hard for a tree that stands by the wayside to keep its fruit till it be ripe.' "[8] University Hospital, as we have seen, affords its physicians some protection so they can adhere to their own high standards for excellence. It gives them time to take pains with examination, with chartwork, with evaluation of findings. The University Hospital atmosphere also supports commitments to continuing search, and belief that there is always hope, always some new finding to extend knowledge as well as life.[9] We have also seen that the atmosphere in University Hospital protects its members somewhat against the pressure to divert their attention toward conveying symbols of authority and symbols of competence as they work in their group with ward patients.[10] In such an enviroment physicians can concentrate on complexities of the medical problem, or on research implications of a finding, even against counter pressures.

It became obvious in observing the house staff at University Hospital that they experienced both social and technical needs to keep abreast of literature. Following this, physicians who prosper in the University Hospital environment have good chances of appointments there or at similar centers where they will continue to be affirmed in a lifetime of learning and exchange with colleagues.

The emphasis on effective action at Community Hospital and the absence of medical students, professors, and other reminders of medical school and education provide comparatively less consistent pressure for continuing education. Also, for the man in private practice "time is money" and beyond that, patients are often impatient with extended deliberation. Through repeated experiences, the physician at Community Hospital sometimes may become more aware of the cost, than of rewards, of quiet deliberation. Indeed, we recall one senior man at Community Hospital saying that some doctors request another laboratory test as an "excuse" for deliberation and postponing a decision. In Community Hospital E where all attending physicians were full time, but at the same time oriented somewhat more to the community of private practice than to the university, some attendings expressed pride over the dispatch with which a thorough diagnostic work-up could be done in their hospital. At the regular early morning specialty conference of house-staff members in this same hospital, new interns were reminded to make their reports brief—and they were interrupted if they began to go into detail. This contrasts with the resident's comment in one university hospital that he appreciated training in his hospital because he could take his time with a patient, and consider many possibilities.

House-staff members at Community Hospital did take time to read and they sometimes complained, as did their colleagues at University Hospital, that they did not have time to keep up with the literature. But in the university-affiliated environment, it seemed that the intern might be more likely to be chided for failing to order some diagnostic test, while in the nonaffiliated hospital, where dispatch was more prized, the intern might be "called" for using one more test as "an excuse" to delay a decision. Probably in the hospital, as in later practice, "I do not have time," may signify something about the priorities of commitments and forecast which of several pressing matters will be the most often postponed in favor of others.

At present, the community hospitals, set aside from academic life may not provide scholarly nurture for local physicians in practice. But they might be in a better position presently than are some academic settings, to provide relevant continuing education in forms that are most likely to be listened to by doctors who must be concerned with efficiency and dispatch. Lindsay Beaton argued effectively for new concepts in education that can keep the solo physician in a meaningful relationship with his own educational parents. He spoke of the situation of the local medical doctor, often without admitting privileges, who "does not find himself totally welcome or befriended by the medical colleges in his task of keeping himself updated . . . The private practitioner has increasingly, therefore, turned to his own devices for modernizing himself, for prolonging his absorption of knowledge. The universities help a little; they send out their circuit-riding professors, they sponsor courses, they contrive superficial but sparkling television shows on esoteric topics. The hospitals and professional associations work harder at the matter. The American Academy of General Practice and the American Psychiatric Association have been perhaps the most assiduous laborers in this vineyard. Some dedicated and very able men have given largely of their time and competence, their energies and their hearts, to such programs. You have heard and will hear this day of isolated successful efforts. But, on the whole, continuing education is too little and too late. And sometimes worse, like Ambrose Bierce's opinion of water as a drink—cheap but not good. Far too often the doctor so enlisted is given only technical information, vocational trade-school gimmicks, not the 'scholarly nurture' he needs and seeks."[11]

The present dichotomy between academicians and practitioners can play a major part in failure to provide relevant programs of continuing education for physicians. When medical schools provide such courses, they may not meet the needs of physicians in the community, in part because the academicians are out of touch with some realities of local practice.

Match and Mismatch

In Chapter III I suggested that a variable worth considering may be the "fit" between the doctor in training and the particular learning environment. Daniel Funkenstein reports Wispe's studies where most students could learn equally well in either highly organized and authoritarian classes, or in permissive and pupil-centered classes. But at the two ends of a personality continuum, the learning of the individual student was related to the interaction between his personality type and the teaching method.[12]

Indicating the need for matching the intellectual climate with medical student, John Caughey wrote, "It is a source of constant astonishment to me how often situations which challenge one student to peak performance and significant professional development seem in another student to undermine his confidence and retard his growth."[13] Not only the intellectual ability and the personality of a student, but also his career plans can influence how he fares in internship. When he fits poorly in his learning environment, the profession's chances of influencing him are probably very much reduced.

Several attributes of University Hospital can contribute to chances for identification within the specialty group and at the same time provide the reinforcements for open discussion, admission of uncertainty, and search for knowledge stimulated in medical school. Conditions of common purpose and similar origins and goals, and sufficient positions in each rank to allow mobility for all aspirants, frequent interaction within the specialty group and limited outside contacts—these can support identification and reinforce commitments to keeping an open mind and can help to train the physician to face and accept uncertainty. For the "proud company" of physicians who have moved successfully through the "best schools" and the "best hospitals" and whose career plans are a good match for the dominant direction of the teaching hospital, the medical educational career can be a smooth and well-articulated sequence. Even when such a medical student goes to a distant affiliated hospital for internship and for residency, the chances are good that he will find some continuity of influence and sometimes even people he knows in circulating ranks of cosmopolitans. But this describes the situation of a small portion of the nation's physicians.[14] We have quoted some who find this sequence alien and impossible to follow.

At the present, some of the other career directions in medicine are less effectively served and the training sequences toward them are less well articulated and less consistent. As the Millis Report suggests, the selection and training for the demanding career of family physician is more a matter of residuals or default than it is a consistent and sustained direction.[15] Going through years of training in a hospital where the more obscure and complex cases are the ones considered "interesting" and where work in an out-patient department is not highly valued, getting accustomed to working mostly with indigent patients is not the optimum in articulated training for a practice with ambulatory middle-class patients who mostly have ordinary medical problems.

We have seen that the selection of internship programs within the large number of community hospitals may be more casual and less well informed than is the selection of just the right place for the more favored student. If a student today takes an internship in a nonaffiliated hospital, he may experience some sharp differences between what he is taught and what is done in medicine. If he takes a rotating internship in a large affiliated hospital that also has straight internships, the generalist or the family-oriented intern may find himself somewhat outside the group of medical house-staff members. Then as he moves to his next assignment, he will be somewhat on the edges of surgery and so on till he has "served his term." The high-morale specialty group may be identified with its specialty service and its chief, and the chief in turn may speak of "his boys," with some proprietary pride. Here, as elsewhere, a tight in-group with good esprit de corps can make the experience of the outsider all the more distressing, and it can be a force making for alienation.

The transient house-staff members, or those poorly matched with their learning environment, without anyone ever intending it, may become the orphans in a series of foster homes in medicine, and they may drift out to the fringes of the medical system somewhat beyond the control of medical colleagues. The specialty group that serves as the protector of some values in medicine at the same time means that physicians who are excluded from such groups and have no other groups to join may be estranged from the medical academy—with unfortunate consequences for the profession and the quality of medical care in the country.[16]

Kenneth Clute, in his study of general practice in Canada and Nova Scotia, found that 28 percent of the physicians in Ontario and a much larger portion in Nova Scotia demonstrated gross inadequacies that gave the evaluation team ". . . grave misgivings [over] deficiencies . . . [which] were thought likely to expose their patients to serious risk."[17] Such findings urge that considered attention be paid to the social function that hospitals and viable continuing education programs can serve beyond the more obvious function of isolated attempts to bring the latest medical advances to the solo practitioner.

Delivery of Health Care

Just as the physician must keep moving ahead in order to keep even with scientific advance, he may also have to advance apace to keep up with rising expectations for care and for delivery of services.

In the first chapter it was noted that the public may suspect that medicine is not doing for it all that it should. Public criticism seems directed at faulty application rather than at basic knowledge and skills. The "fault," it is suggested, is in interpersonal and interprofessional rather than in poor physical techniques.[18] American medicine is not alone in having produced medical advances that then spur expectations and criticisms. For example, a *New York Times* headline (September 8, 1968) reads, "Soviet Physicians Said to Lack Bedside Manner." While some of the criticism, here as elsewhere, may be counted as a consequence of ambivalence, some of it may reflect the outcome of the repeated experiences fostered in some learning environments.

One spokesman for the patient's perspective suggests that nurses, as well as doctors, sometimes cloak their work in mystery, perhaps without planning it:

> It seems to me that many persons in medicine today continue to foster and cherish mystery for mystery's sake. I am thinking of the prescriptions still written illegibly in pig-Latin. I am thinking of the enigmatic smile after the blood pressure readings, and the utter silence after the retinal blood vessels are examined. I am thinking of the nurse's solid mask after the removal of the thermometer from wherever it was . . . Doubtless, many patients must be diminished to be made manageable or even tolerable, but diminishing the stroke patient is risky business, for he has already been diminished by Act of God and in addition to his neurologic symptoms, he is full of fear—raw, elemental fear—not necessarily of death but of incapacity or destitution. From whom is he going to draw the courage without which he will not truly recover? Not from a silent practitioner; not from a stuffy practitioner; not from a practitioner, whether doctor, therapist or nurse, who is aloof. He will draw courage as he perceives human understanding underlying the professional technics of those into whose care he has been given.[19]

Others, equally eloquent on medical faculties, speak of the importance of attention to the frightened person who is a patient. Still, the social structures of some hospital learning-environments provide frequent and easy means for legitimized escape from having to acknowledge and take hold of responsibility for attempting to help the patient manage his fears and losses. There are probably adequate controls over the knowledge and technical skills a medical graduate must have, but as John Caughey observes, the nonintellectual components of medical education which are of critical importance do not receive the attention they should have.[20] Less well specified, less well developed are the environmental conditions in hospitals that will best contribute to the education of physicians in community medicine. Many avenues of fruitful investigation toward improvements in the health care system beckon research. There is recurring evidence that patients can and do help each other effectively, yet the medical care system seldom takes this potential into account.[21]

We know that a professional label is not a necessary predictor of the actual authority and functions of individuals in complex organizations.[22] The physician should be able to command prestige and respect—and necessary compliance with medical advice—wherever he works. But it may often be left up to his ability to negotiate before his legislative claim will be accepted. Yet little attention is paid to how learning environments can influence the development of physicians' ability to establish the most efficacious relationships with other professionals. Relatively little attention is given to the matter of how hospital environments can facilitate learning about the doctor-patient relationship, and how to increase compliance with necessary medical advice.

Much is said about fragmentation and duplication of effort. Much is written about the need for comprehensive care. Physicians and economists discuss the waste of energy, time and money inherent in duplication. Peter Lee described a study of the records of all patients whose charts weighed one pound and more where it was found that the majority of these patients had functional complaints and were being shuttled from one specialty clinic to another. "It was evident that this type of symptomatic management of patients with emotional problems was uneconomical, inhumane, and ineffective. By spending more time with these patients during visits to the comprehensive medicine clinic, it was possible in most cases to define the basic nature of their problem, and in a great many cases to effect significant

improvement in personal well-being and social effectiveness
. . . the comprehensive approach and the spending of adequate
time with each patient was in the long run an economical procedure."[23] Efforts at such clinics are promising. Yet, little is
being done to study social structure and value climates in hospitals generally to discover what patterns of rewards and sanction
allow fragmentation as a part of daily reality in house-staff training. The social structure and value climate may be the "message"
that either supports or subverts lectures on the priority of comprehensive care.

I have described some aspects of the two cultures in medicine,
each sustained by its own type of hospital and extended by the
structure of its own medical practice. A third is beginning to
compete successfully for recruits, funds, and other resources in
medicine as articles, books, hours of curriculum time, grants
and research funds have increasingly related to community
health.[24] Presently, the ethos of community medicine is closely
related to medical school and the behavioral sciences—in some
places more closely than it relates to the community of local
practitioners. At first, it seems paradoxical that the local physicians, whose primary work and experience and skill relates
directly to the lay community, are probably among the physicians
farthest away from both planning and effecting community
health efforts for the future.[25] Both the men in community
medicine and the practitioners who treat mostly ambulatory
patients work with people who are relatively free to follow medical advice or to ignore it, and they thus share problems that the
physician in University Hospital may sometimes miss in his work
with selected patients on hospital wards.

But the paradox is less marked when we see that the paths of
community medicine and solo practice are divergent. The relationship between patient and *the* doctor is the lodestar of private practice; but in community medicine the team and the
hospital become involved in cooperative efforts on behalf of patients. There may be many "third parties" as the team works
in the large organization to pull together the work of many specialists and sometimes many agencies on behalf of all people who
need it in a community. The patient sometimes in turn tends

to become loyal to the hospital, the doctors, the clinic. For patients with chronic illness, many interns and residents will come and go, but the clinic, the hospital endures.

In Chapter VIII, I discussed the different criteria that patients and physicians use to judge medical competence. Doctors may sometimes assume even larger differences than the facts support, particularly when the patients are part of a clinic population. An incidental finding in one study of ambulatory patients on welfare was that patients' appraisals of physicians' performance did "correlate highly with professional criteria for assessing likelihood of competent professional performance."[26]

In contrast to perpetuating an air of mystery, the physicians in community medicine may strive to reduce the mystery of disease and to encourage and "educate" a population toward more rational patterns around health.[27] Then too, while the patient comes to the doctor in private practice, the health team goes out to the community in preventive efforts and moves to bring patients into clinics. The physician in private practice may be repelled at the suggestion of "advertising for patients" but the community medicine program may advertise to bring people to a mobile chest X-ray unit and to come in for Pap tests. Persuasion in the form of calls and reminders and posters and handbills to draw the attention of "target groups" fit in with the goals and commitments of community medicine. But these same actions do violence to the ethos held with near reverence by many private practitioners.

The acts that the educator in community medicine sees as progress toward large health goals, the man in solo practice may see as subversive of the very essentials of the system to which he is committed. The final incendiary social fact in the antipathy of local doctors to a program in community medicine, may be that they sometimes direct their efforts toward some of the same patients.

Improved interchange between local practitioners, the community hospitals, and the men of community medicine in teaching centers could benefit the larger concern of medicine—not only by increasing chances to upgrade local practice. Such exchange between teaching centers and community hospitals may sometimes also mean that innovative moves which the flexible structures of some community hospitals may best contribute are not lost to medical education. The physicians in community hospitals publish relatively infrequently, and tend not to be heard from or listened to within medical education. As DuVal notes, "Those whose orientation has been primarily inside the academic sphere are often surprised, albeit unwarranted, that so many sound ideas about medical education can arise from thoughtful members of the profession who are outside the school."[28]

There may be an increasing need for the "social scientist physician" described by Funkenstein, who would have knowledge of the complex organizations, community structure, and functions that physicians ordinarily lack.[29] As Cecil Sheps and his committee report: "Although it is understandable, and oftentimes even desirable for the individual professor to be single-minded and dedicated to his research and teaching, it is the study group's opinion that it is most regrettable, if not unforgivable, for hospitals affiliated with medical schools to be less than fully aware of their broad responsibilities toward the goal of community service."[30]

Community hospitals, suitably supported, encouraged, and related to the whole enterprise of medical education, may provide one vehicle for the development and support of community health efforts. These hospitals are more likely to be accustomed to coping with some of the exigencies of the relationships between local practitioners and hospitals, the press, the public, and the local political structure. Such hospitals may also be less forbidding to the practitioner and thus in the best position to influence him toward better practice. The structures of many of the community hospitals are flexible and therefore able to allow individual innovative efforts to solve problems, and to make necessary accommodations to needs within the individual community.

It would seem that a consideration of the different functions that a variety of hospitals serve may be in order before heroic efforts are bent either toward transferring all the approved programs in community hospitals into small university hospitals, or to make drastic changes in the university-affiliated hospitals to make them more pleasing to the layman and his criteria for evaluation—when those changes might undermine other values, other patterns.

We have seen something of the disparity in the professional lives of physicians who are far apart, each working in his own culture. Many people have already decried some ill effects of the split. The "cosmopolitan" men in the medical school context tend to be oriented to their discipline, their specialist colleagues in the university centers, and to the granting agencies of the country. The public needs such physicians trained in environments that reinforce and protect the physician's commitment to admitting uncertainty and to extending knowledge.

In contrast, the solo practitioners tend to be more oriented toward local patients and local problems, and they may be fearful of change imposed from the outside and resentful of any intrusion into the relationship. But local communities need hospital services near at hand, and local physicians need hospitals for their facilities as well as for the chances for discourse with other physicians and for practice-oriented continuing education. Such physicians need stimulus to keep them abreast of advances and the means to facilitate their effort. The work also needs mechanisms to provide visibility by colleagues.

The public wants scientific advance, but it also wants to believe that its physicians are primarily directed toward the individual person. It wants to be reassured and treated with respect by its physicians. "Somewhere between the proposition that the customer is always right and the proposition that the public be damned must be an uneasy Aristotelian mean, and toward this the concept of professional need for medical care . . . uneasily steers itself."[31]

Notes

Index

Notes

INTRODUCTION

1. Citizens Commission on Graduate Medical Education, *The Graduate Education of Physicians* (Chicago: American Medical Association, 1966), pp. 9–10. William E. Sedlacek, "Attitudes of Residents toward Their Complex Role in Medical Education," *Journal of Medical Education*, 43 (1968), 344–348.

2. Abraham Flexner, *Medical Education in the United States and Canada* (New York: Carnegie Foundation, 1910).

3. Maurice Levin, "Self-Scrutiny in the Discussion of Medical Education," working paper, Conference on Psychiatry and Medical Education, Washington, D.C., November 1966, Serial No. 26.

4. Samuel W. Bloom, "The Sociology of Medical Education: Some Comments on the State of a Field," *Milbank Memorial Fund Quarterly*, 43 (1965), 143–184; Harold J. Simon, "Social and Behavioral Sciences in Medical Education," *Journal of Medical Education*, 41 (1966) 1049–1056; Mervyn Susser, "Teaching Social Medicine in the United States," *Milbank Memorial Fund Quarterly*, 44 (1966), 389–413; John C. Donovan and Curtis J. Lund, "Internships in a University Department of Obstetrics-Gynecology: A Comparative Study," *Journal of Medical Education*, 43 (1968), 48–54; Willard C. Rappleye, "Future of the Non-University Affiliated Municipal and Voluntary Hospitals," paper presented at the Meeting of the American College of Surgeons, Bronx Chapter, May 1960; Dale N. Schumacher, "An Analysis of Student Clinical Activities," *Journal of Medical Education*, 43 (1968), 383–388.

5. Lowell T. Coggeshall, *Planning for Medical Progress through Education* (Evanston, Ill.: Association of American Medical Colleges, 1965), p. 39.

6. Medical educators have explored the possibilities of differences in performance on National Boards of Interns going to and coming from different hospitals. One group found that university-affiliated hospitals obtained interns who did better on the boards than did interns going to nonaffiliated

hospitals and noted that affiliated hospitals with more than 75 percent of their positions filled turned out interns who did better on the National Boards. *See* Edithe J. Levit, Charles F. Schumacher, and John P. Hubbard, "The Internship," *Journal of the American Medical Association,* 189 (1964), 299–305.

The relatively meager number of studies of interns and residents by sociologists is surprising since sociologists claim that an intensive and extended training period can have profound influence on the developing professional. The molding power of first impressions is a theme of some interesting work in psychology and sociology. *See,* for example, Theodore M. Newcomb, *Social Psychology* (New York: Dryden Press, 1950), pp. 199–207. And *see* Karl Mannheim's discussion of the impact of first experiences in "The Problem of Generations," *Essays on the Sociology of Knowledge* (New York: Oxford University Press, 1952), pp. 296–299. But a 1962 bibliography in medical sociology listed eighteen titles on medical education; none of these specifically related to interns, residents, or their training programs. *See* Eliot Freidson, "The Sociology of Medicine," *Current Sociology,* 10–11 (1961–1962), 168–169. The 1964 *Cumulative Book Index* reports several works on medical students, yet nothing on interns or residents. In 1965 the New York Public Library catalogue had no entries for the subjects, intern or resident, either separately or as a subhead under medicine, hospitals, or education. (*Intern,* the anonymously authored diary of an intern's experience that soared to best-seller heights, had yet to be catalogued.) The Library of Congress had only eight entries on interns or residents. But each of these was a product of physicians' efforts, not the work of social scientists.

There are, of course, a few scattered works on the intern and resident in sociological journals, but most of them date from 1960 on. For example, Morris J. Daniels, "Affect and Its Control in the Medical Intern," *American Journal of Sociology,* 66 (1960), 259–267; Melvin Seeman and John W. Evans, "Stratification and Hospital Care: I. The Performance of the Medical Interne," *American Sociological Review,* 26 (1961), 67–80.

Columbia University's Bureau of Applied Social Research began to turn its attention to the intern and residency phase of medical education by 1958. The doctoral dissertation that provides the background for this report and one other completed one in progress are out of that study, supported by a grant-in-aid from The Commonwealth Fund. There were numerous studies, published and unpublished, from the Bureau's study of medical students. *See,* for example, Robert K. Merton, George G. Reader, and Patricia L. Kendall, eds., *The Student-Physician* (Cambridge, Mass.: Harvard University Press, 1957).

7. Samuel W. Bloom, "The Process of Becoming a Physician," *Annals of the American Academy of Political and Social Science,* 346 (1963), 87, reprint edition.

8. Leland S. McKittrick, "Rational Responses to Graduate Education of Physicians," *Journal of the American Medical Association,* 201 (1967), 112.

9. This study was conducted by the Bureau of Applied Social Research of Columbia University under a grant-in-aid from The Commonwealth Fund. *See* "Proposal for a Comparative Study of the Internship and Residency: To The Commonwealth Fund," Bureau of Applied Social Research of Columbia University, April 1958.

10. The perceptions of interns when they first arrive may be similar to the "first-day insights" that some sociologists have noticed. Blanche Geer wrote: "Participant-observers sometimes say that the major themes of a study appeared very early in the field of work, although they may have been unrecognized . . . the answer to the question, 'Do strategies and concepts change in the first days of field work?' is emphatically *yes*. Furthermore, many of the changes are of such a nature as to affect subsequent field work radically" (Blanche Geer, "First Days in the Field," in Phillip E. Hammond, ed., *Sociologists at Work* [New York: Basic Books, 1964], pp. 337, 340). A personal communication from Rose Coser comments on her similar experience with field work and also mentions Renée Fox's similar experience.

11. The "town and gown" phrase occurs in discussions of several professions. In medicine, it refers to the great differences between the work, training, orientation, and culture of people who are local practitioners versus those in full time academic medicine. C. P. Snow's "Two Cultures" relates to the divergence between the culture of town and gown.

These interviews were conducted as part of a study of the relation between medical educators and medical practitioners, by the Bureau of Applied Social Research of Columbia University, under the direction of Patricia L. Kendall, for the 1962 Teaching Institute of the Association of American Medical Colleges. For a report of that study, *see* Patricia L. Kendall, *The Relationship Between Medical Educators and Medical Practitioners: Sources of Strain and Occasions for Cooperation* (Evanston, Ill.: Association of American Medical Colleges, 1965).

12. Claire Selltiz, Marie Jahoda, Morton Deutsch, and Stuart W. Cook, *Research Methods in Social Relations*, rev. ed. (New York: Holt, Rinehart, and Winston, 1959), pp. 207–221. Rue Bucher also found informal comments useful in observation; *see* "The Psychiatric Residency and Professional Socialization," *Journal of Health and Human Behavior*, 6 (1965), 197–206.

13. This figure of 195 does not include psychiatric residents. The nationwide study concerned itself with programs in the four services: medicine, surgery, obstetrics-gynecology, and pediatrics—services routinely included in rotating internships. Barton and Lazarsfeld cite the potential usefulness of written-in comments as clues for analysis. *See* Allen H. Barton and Paul F. Lazarsfeld, "Some Functions of Qualitative Analysis in Social Research," *Frankfurter Beitrage Zur Soziologie*, 1 (1955), 321–361.

14. Lipset, Trow, and Coleman suggest that their effective access route to individual shops in their study of the International Typographical Union came through the union representatives and indicate something of authority

relationships in print shops. *See* Seymour M. Lipset, Martin A. Trow, and James S. Coleman, *Union Democracy* (Glencoe, Ill.: The Free Press, 1956), p. 25. In a somewhat similar way, Whyte entered the Italian-American community under the auspices of Doc, a key member of a gang, whose support seemed significant in Whyte's acceptance by Doc's followers as well as by members of other related gangs. *See* William F. Whyte, *Street Corner Society* (Chicago: University of Chicago Press, 1943).

15. Entree into Community Hospital through an attending physician and the administrator may resemble the dual entree into a community which was used in Merton's housing study and in Babchuk and Goode's study of a selling group. Although first approval came from the attending physician, the final okay and ready assistance during the course of study at Community Hospital did come primarily from the administration. *See* Robert K. Merton, "Selected Problems of Field Work in the Planned Community," *American Sociological Review,* 12 (1947), 304–312; and Nicholas Babchuk and William J. Goode, "Work Incentives in a Self-Determined Group," *American Sociological Review,* 16 (1951), 679–687.

16. "It may, on occasion, be better to let influential persons in the community handle the explanation of the investigator's work" (Selltiz *et al., Research Methods,* p. 220).

17. Rose Laub Coser, *Life in the Ward* (East Lansing: Michigan State University Press, 1962), p. xix.

18. Kenneth F. Clute, *The General Practitioner: A Study of Medical Education in Ontario and Nova Scotia* (Toronto: University of Toronto Press, 1963), p. 18. Morton Deutsch found that students, when they were observed in a situation in which they were cooperating, seemed less aware of observers than students who were in competition. *See* "An Experimental Study of the Effects of Cooperation and Competition upon Group Process," *Human Relations,* 2 (1949), 199–231.

19. William Foote Whyte, "Observational Field-Work Methods," in Marie Jahoda, Morton Deutsch, and Stuart W. Cook, eds., *Research Methods in Social Relations,* part 2 (New York: Dryden Press, 1951), pp. 493–513. And *see* Selltiz *et al., Research Methods,* pp. 200–234.

20. Elaine and John Cumming suggest some of the unfortunate consequences that can develop when researchers do not attend carefully enough to emerging—often erroneous—definitions of the "purpose" of the work in the field. *See* Elaine Cumming and John Cumming, *Closed Ranks* (Cambridge, Mass.: Harvard University Press, 1957).

21. *Ibid.,* pp. 36–48.

22. Renée Fox, in her study of a metabolic research ward in a teaching hospital, came to a similar decision. "I felt that it would be wiser to appear on the ward as the sociologist I actually was than to assume a form of camouflage" (Renée C. Fox, *Experiment Perilous* [Glencoe, Ill.: The Free Press, 1959], p. 213).

23. Deutsch's observation was that people in groups observed over time

seemed to become less aware of the observer's presence. See Deutsch, "An Experimental Study." *See also* Alvin Zander, "Systematic Observation of Small Face-to-Face Groups," in Jahoda *et al., Research Methods,* pp. 515–538.

24. Peter M. Blau, "The Research Process in the Study of the Dynamics of Bureaucracy," in Phillip E. Hammond, ed., *Sociologists at Work* (New York: Basic Books, 1964), p. 28.

25. William J. Goode and Paul K. Hatt, "Observation," in *Methods in Social Research* (New York: McGraw-Hill Book Co., 1952), pp. 122–123.

26. Don D. Smith, "Cognitive Consistency and the Perception of Others' Opinions," *Public Opinion Quarterly,* 32 (1968), 1–15. Among the many studies of selective perception, attention, and recall, see the following: Harry Stack Sullivan, *The Interpersonal Theory of Psychiatry,* Helen Swick Perry and Mary Ladd Gawel, eds. (New York: W. W. Norton, 1953), pp. 319–320, 333–334, 367–384, and *passim;* Jerome S. Bruner, "Personality Dynamics and the Process of Perceiving," in Robert R. Blake and Glenn V. Ramsey, eds., *Perception: An Approach to Personality* (New York: Ronald Press, 1951), pp. 121–147; Jerome M. Levine and Gardner Murphy, "The Learning and Forgetting of Controversial Material," in Eleanor E. Maccoby, Theodore M. Newcomb, and Eugene L. Hartley, eds., *Readings in Social Psychology* (New York: Henry Holt and Co., 1958), pp. 94–101.

27. "The best time for recording is undoubtedly on the spot and during the event. This results in a minimum of selective bias and distortion through memory . . . However the observer records his immediate impressions, he should write up, as soon as possible after a period of observation, a complete account of everything in the situation that he wishes to remember . . . increase the objectivity of his observations by indicating, as he writes up his notes, which statements refer to actual events and which represent his interpretations" (Selltiz *et al., Research Methods,* pp. 210–211, 214).

28. Merton, discussing field work for the Craftown study, suggests, "The outsider has 'stranger value.' For just as temporary boon companions on an ocean voyage will exchange the most private confidences, precisely because they will probably never meet again, so the unattached field observer will have access to confidences which will not be made known to members of a management staff. When there is little prospect of continued contact, there is less sense of self-exposure" (Merton, "Selected Problems," p. 305).

29. *See* Robert K. Merton, Marjorie Fiske, and Patricia L. Kendall, *The Focused Interview* (Glencoe, Ill.: The Free Press, 1956); Paul F. Lazarsfeld, "The Controversy over Detailed Interviews: An Offer for Negotiation," *Public Opinion Quarterly,* 8 (1944), 38–60; and Selltiz *et al,, Research Methods,* pp. 263–268.

30. H. H. Gerth and C. Wright Mills, trans. and eds., *From Max Weber: Essays in Sociology* (New York: Oxford University Press, 1946), pp. 59–61; Max Weber, *The Methodology of the Social Sciences,* trans. E. A. Shils and H. A. Finch (Glencoe, Ill.: The Free Press, 1949), pp. 89–105 and *passim.*

Goode's comment is appropriate for working with any typology: "The purpose of a theoretical concept is to allow us to continue our analysis, not to stop it" (William J. Goode, *After Divorce* [Glencoe, Ill.: The Free Press, 1956], p. 88).

31. Julien Freund, *The Sociology of Max Weber* (New York: Pantheon Books, 1968), p. 8.

I. TRENDS IN MEDICAL PRACTICE AND TRAINING

1. Alexis de Tocqueville, *Democracy in America,* trans. Henry Reeve (New York: Schocken Books, 1961), II, 153.

2. Walter J. McNerney, "Comprehensive Personal Health Care Services: A Management Challenge to the Health Professions," *American Journal of Public Health,* 57 (1967), 1717–1727. *See also* John H. Knowles, *The Teaching Hospital,* "Introduction," pp. 1–6, and "Medical School, Teaching Hospital, and Social Responsibility," pp. 84–145 (Cambridge, Mass.: Harvard University Press, 1966). The same trend shows up in medical education. *See* Resources Analysis Branch, Office of Program Planning, National Institutes of Health, *Manpower for Medical Research 1965–1970,* Report No. 3 (January 1963). "For the first time in the eight years that this information has been collected, the percentage of full-time faculty receiving all or part of their support from federal research and/or training grants declined" (Council on Medical Education, "Medical Education," *Journal of the American Medical Association,* 202 [1967], 749–750).

3. As Robert Ebert puts it, "The more affluent a society becomes, the more concern there is for individual health, and the greater is the desire to maintain physical health. Sickness and death are no longer accepted as inevitable, and the public comes to look upon medical care as a right and not a privilege. In particular, there are reluctances to accept medical care as charity" (Robert H. Ebert, "The Dilemma of Medical Teaching in an Affluent Society," in Knowles, *The Teaching Hospital,* p. 69). Titmuss affirms the influence of society's value commitments on health behavior: "the larger the investment by any society in 'individualism' . . . the more may 'health consciousness' spread . . . as society becomes more health conscious . . . the more may each individual become dependent . . . in an age of scientific medicine on other individuals . . . The high esteem of psychology and science in the American culture both emphasizes and expresses this sense of dependency in the search for good health. In relative terms, the individual may come to feel more dependent on psychotherapy, on medical science, on doctors; less on his own inner resources" (Richard M. Titmuss, *Essays on 'The Welfare State'* [London: George Allen & Unwin Ltd., 1958], p. 134).

4. Walter Goodman, "The Doctor's Image Is Sickly," *New York Times Magazine,* October 16, 1966. Goodman notes that the doctor is still very

near the top in prestige, ranking just below Supreme Court justices, but then goes on to point out a wide range of symptoms of public discontent with doctors. Goodman states that Martin L. Gross, in *The Doctors*, "notifies us early [that the modern physician] has become 'one of man's most potent killers and cripplers' and he does not let us forget it for the next 560 pages" (Walter Goodman, review in *New York Times Book Week*, October 2, 1966, p. 4).

For some other books that feed discontent with or "unmask" the doctors, see Richard Carter, *The Doctor Business* (Garden City, N.Y.: Doubleday, 1958); Selig Greenberg, *The Troubled Calling* (New York: Macmillan Company, 1965); Louis Lasagna, *The Doctors' Dilemmas* (New York: Collier Books, 1963); Doctor X, *Intern* (New York: Harper & Row, 1965); Roul Tunley, *The American Health Scandal* (New York: Harper & Row, 1966).

5. Robert K. Merton and Elinor Barber, "Sociological Ambivalence," in Edward A. Tiryakian, ed., *Sociological Theory, Values, and Sociocultural Change* (New York: The Free Press of Glencoe, 1963), p. 108.

6. William A. Gamson and Howard Suchman, "Some Undercurrents in the Prestige of Physicians," *American Journal of Sociology*, 68 (1963), 463–470.

7. David Riesman, *The Story of Medicine in the Middle Ages* (New York: Paul B. Hoeber, 1935), especially pp. 365–366.

8. C. Joseph Stetler and Alan R. Moritz, *Doctor and Patient and the Law* (St. Louis: C. V. Mosby Company, 1962), pp. 441–442.

9. *See* Ebert, "The Dilemma of Medical Teaching," pp. 66–83; U.S. Department of Health, Education, and Welfare, "Hill-Burton Program: State Plan Data for Hospitals and Related Medical Facilities" (Washington, D.C.: Public Health Service Publication, No. 930-F-2, revised 1963), p. 21; E. Richard Weinerman, "Yale Studies in Ambulatory Medical Care," *New England Journal of Medicine*, 272 (1965), 953; Division of Operational Studies of the AAMC, "Full Time Medical School Faculty," *Journal of Medical Education*, 41 (1966), 297–298; Richard Harris, "Annals of Legislation: Medicare," *The New Yorker*, July 2, 1966, p. 34; and Milton I. Roemer, "The Future of Social Medicine in the United States," p. 13, paper presented at the Annual Meeting of the American Sociological Association, Miami Beach, Florida, August 1966. The Council on Medical Education has reported that "Since 1960–1961, there has been an increase in full-time faculty of 8,185, or 74%, over the 11,111 reported for that year. The clinical faculty has almost doubled, increasing by 87%, while the basic science faculty has grown by 50% in the same period" ("Medical Education," pp. 746–747).

10. "The field of general practice continued to decline in terms of new trainees, since the proportion of filled positions fell to 48%, a decline of 11% from that of the previous year. Foreign graduates held 67% of the positions filled in general practice" (Council on Medical Education, "Med-

ical Education," p. 770). *See also* George Rosen, "The Impact of Hospital on the Physician, the Patient and Community," *Hospital Administration,* 9 (1964), 15–33.

11. Fremont J. Lyden, H. Jack Geiger, and Osler L. Peterson, *The Training of Good Physicians: Critical Factors in Career Choices* (Cambridge, Mass.: Harvard University Press, 1968).

12. Council on Medical Education, "Medical Education," p. 778.

13. Articles that have brought medical education to public attention include items such as Martin Tolchin, "Hospitals Find Interns Scarce," *New York Times,* March 15, 1966, p. 41, and the one on Harvard Medical School in *Life,* May 18, 1962, pp. 84–94; and Doctor X, *Intern.* Among the several studies that find more recent medical school graduates to be better trained, *see* Paul L. Sanazaro and John W. Williamson, "A Classification of Physician Performance in Internal Medicine," *Journal of Medical Education,* 43 (1968), 389–397.

Some of the schools that Flexner visited claimed no entrance requirements, and justified indiscriminate recruitment as "help" for the poor youths of the country. *See* Abraham Flexner, *Medical Education in the United States and Canada,* a report to the Carnegie Foundation for the Advancement of Teaching (New York: Carnegie Foundation, 1910), p. xi. The miscellany of proprietary schools, some innocent of affiliation with university or hospitals, moved to the realm of historical oddities after the Flexner report and action by the profession. But in those not so distant days, a few schools and some of the "better ones" demanded only a high school diploma for entry. The medical school diploma was a license to practice. "The examinations, brief, oral, and secret, plucked almost none at all . . . The man who had settled his tuition bill was thus practically assured of his degree, whether he had regularly attended lectures or not" (Abraham Flexner, *I Remember* [New York: Simon and Schuster, 1940], p. 119). *See also* Abraham Flexner, *Medical Education, A Comparative Study* (New York: Macmillan Company, 1925). These surveys of medical education from not much more than a half century ago in this country should be required reading for anyone who feels "things have never been worse."

John S. Billings in his opening address at the Johns Hopkins Hospital in 1889 estimated that "not more than 5 percent of medical graduates have any opportunities worth speaking of to study and treat diseases in the living man when they receive their diplomas" (Alan M. Chesney, *The Johns Hopkins Hospital and the Johns Hopkins University School of Medicine* [Baltimore: The Johns Hopkins Press, 1943], I, 247).

Some indication of competition among foreign medical school graduates to obtain intern and residency training positions here can be seen in a recent decision of the Board of Trustees of the Education Council for Foreign Medical Graduates which "announced that after March, 1964, examination, the granting of temporary certificates would be abolished. The certificates previously issued will entitle their holders, in some instances, to continue in graduate training until June 30, 1966, but with the October 21, 1964, examination and thereafter, candidates must score 75 or more in order to qualify for eligibility for certification" (*Journal of the American Medical Education*, 190 [1964], 632).

14. *See* Everett Cherrington Hughes, "Dilemmas and Contradictions of Status," in Lewis A. Coser and Bernard Rosenberg, eds., *Sociological Theory* (New York: Macmillan Company, 1957), pp. 366–376; and Stanley Lieberson, "Ethnic Groups and the Practice of Medicine," *American Sociological Review*, 23 (1958), 542–549. The symbols that patients use may be changing, and would be expected to change with the times.

Binger, commenting on the psychological basis of potentially disturbed communication between physicians and patients, wrote, "What appears to us to be the truth may, when pyramided by anxiety, become to our patients a distorted phantasmagoria" (Carl Binger, *The Doctor's Job* [New York: W. W. Norton & Co., 1945], p. 48). *See also* the study of expectation and communication gaps between physicians and patients by Marion S. Lesser and Vera R. Keane, *Nurse-Patient Relationships in a Hospital Maternity Service* (St. Louis: C. V. Mosby Co., 1956); and Otto Von Mering, "Value Dilemmas and Reciprocally Evoked Transactions of Patient and Curer," *Psychoanalysis and the Psychoanalytic Review*, 49 (1962), 119–143.

15. *See* "What Good Doctors Can Do About Bad Ones," *Medical Economics*, August 14, 1961, pp. 101–148; and "New Legal Rulings Threaten MDs," *Medical World News*, June 22, 1962, pp. 30, 32.

16. James Bordley, III, "Effect of House Staff Training Programs on Patient Care," *Journal of the American Medical Association*, 173 (1960), 1316.

17. Osler L. Peterson, Leon P. Andrews, Robert S. Spain, and Bernard G. Greenberg, "An Analytical Study of North Carolina General Practice, 1953–1954," *Journal of Medical Education*, 31 (1956), part 2, p. 130.

18. Oliver Wendell Holmes, "The Young Practitioner," in William H. Davenport, ed., *The Good Physician* (New York: Macmillan Company, 1962), p. 176.

19. It would be interesting to pursue the variety of such terms employed by each profession and to determine the nature of actions covered by the terms. Would these and other epithets highlight the degree of disparity between the prestige referents and reward systems of each particular profession and its clients, as well as some of the specific problem areas? Merton wrote, "The diagnostic significance of such linguistic indices as epithets has scarcely been explored by the sociologist. Sumner properly observes that epithets produce 'summary criticisms' and definitions of social situations. Dollard also notes that 'epithets frequently define the central issues in a society,' and Sapir has rightly emphasized the importance of context of situations in appraising the significance of epithets . . . A sociological study of 'vocabularies of encomium and opprobrium' should lead to valuable

findings" (Robert K. Merton, *Social Theory and Social Structure* [Glencoe, Ill.: The Free Press, 1957], p. 204, note 24).

Peter Blau, in discussing bureaucracies, observed, "It is well known that a professional jargon helps to unite a group and to set it apart from strangers . . . distinct terms tend to develop in areas of conflict with outsiders, where a reminder of group cohesion is most needed to sustain the individual" (Peter M. Blau, *The Dynamics of Bureaucracy* [Chicago: University of Chicago Press, 1955], p. 88).

20. *See* discussions of change and improvement when communication channels were cleared in a mental hospital, in Alfred H. Stanton and Morris S. Schwartz, *The Mental Hospital* (New York: Basic Books, 1954), pp. 193–243. *See also* a discussion of some reported results of limited cognitive communication of the staff of a psychiatric ward in William Caudill, "Social Processes in a Collective Disturbance on a Psychiatric Ward," in Milton Greenblatt, Daniel J. Levinson, and Richard H. Williams, eds., *The Patient and the Mental Hospital* (Glencoe, Ill.: The Free Press, 1957), pp. 438–471. For a reconsideration of these assumptions *see* Amitai Etzioni, "Interpersonal and Structural Factors in the Study of Mental Hospitals," *Psychiatry*, 23 (1960), 13–22.

21. David Riesman, "Toward an Anthropological Science of Law and the Legal Profession," *American Journal of Sociology*, 57 (1951), 121–135.

22. Everett Cherrington Hughes, "Mistakes at Work," in *Men and Their Work* (Glencoe, Ill.: The Free Press, 1958), pp. 88–101; and Erving Goffman, *The Presentation of Self in Everyday Life* (Garden City, N.Y.: Doubleday Anchor Books, 1959), pp. 45, 70 and *passim*.

23. *See* Talcott Parsons and Renée C. Fox, "Illness, Therapy and the Modern Urban American Family," in E. Gartly Jaco, ed., *Patients, Physicians and Illness* (Glencoe, Ill.: The Free Press, 1958), pp. 234–245.

24. Citizens Commission on Graduate Medical Education, *The Graduate Education of Physicians* (Chicago: American Medical Association, 1966), pp. 48–56 and *passim*.

25. American Medical Association, *Directory of Approved Internships and Residencies* (1967–1968), p. 4, and Table 5, p. 5. *See also* Robert J. Glaser, "The Teaching Hospital and the Medical School," in Knowles, *The Teaching Hospital*, pp. 7–37.

26. "Consolidated List of Hospitals," in AMA, *Directory of Approved Internships*, pp. 31–76, and Table 5, p. 5.

27. Raymond S. Duff and August B. Hollingshead, *Sickness and Society* (New York: Harper & Row, 1968), pp. 124–150.

28. "A Sample Index Based on 17 Per Cent of the Research Grants Awarded in Fiscal Year 1961," Research Grants Index, U.S. Department of Health, Education, and Welfare, Public Health Service (Bethesda, Md.: National Institutes of Health, Division of Research Grants).

29. AMA, *Directory of Approved Internships*, p. 4, Table 5, p. 5, and see Table 2 above.

30. Association of American Medical Colleges, "National Intern and Resident Matching Program, 1958–1968," *Journal of Medical Education,* 43 (1968), 765; and Council on Medical Education, "Medical Education," p. 768.

31. John J. Butler and Jerald T. Hage, "Physician Attitudes toward a Hospital Program in Medical Education," *Journal of Medical Education,* 41 (1966), 913–914.

32. Calculated from "Consolidated List of Hospitals," in AMA, *Directory of Approved Internships,* pp. 63–64.

33. "The medical schools reported major affiliations with 182 hospitals not owned by the schools. On the other hand, 256 hospitals not owned by medical schools reported major affiliations with these schools. In other words, 74 hospitals reported major affiliations that are not recognized as major by the schools" (Cecil G. Sheps, Dean A. Clark, John W. Gerdes, Ethelmarie Halpern, and Nathan Hershey, "Medical Schools and Hospitals: Interdependence for Education and Service," *Journal of Medical Education,* 40 [1965], part 2, p. 17).

34. AMA, *Directory of Approved Internships,* Table 2, p. 2.

35. Alfred North Whitehead, cited in Paul R. Miller, *Sense and Symbol* (New York: Hoeber Medical Division, Harper & Row, 1967), p. 286.

36. AAM Colleges, "National Intern," pp. 764–765; AMA, *Directory of Approved Internships,* p. 17, and Table 10, p. 8.

37. *See* Howard S. Becker and Blanche Geer, "The Fate of Idealism in Medical School," in E. Gartly Jaco, ed., *Patients, Physicians and Illness* (Glencoe, Ill.: The Free Press, 1958), pp. 300–307; Samuel W. Bloom, "The Process of Becoming a Physician," *Annals of the American Academy of Political and Social Science,* 346 (1963), 77–87, reprint edition. Leonard D. Eron notes that "although freshman law students profess to significantly more cynical attitudes by far than do freshman medical students, the seniors in these same schools are equal in the extent of cynical attitude expressed" ("The Effect of Medical Education on Attitudes: A Follow-Up Study," *Journal of Medical Education,* 33 [1958], part 2, p. 27). "The initial enthusiasm and humanistic motivation of fledgling medical students, fresh from the liberal arts, are frequently smothered" (Irving L. Schwartz, "Graduate Education and Medical Education: A Synergism," *Journal of The Mount Sinai Hospital,* 34 [1967], 242). "It is my impression that during the first year and during most of the second year students are receptive of psychiatry, but that some time in the second year this receptiveness diminishes" (William T. Lhamon, personal communication, March 1964). "Junior physicians, however, are more likely to note the importance of interpersonal skills. Sixty-three per cent of the junior physicians and only 42 per cent of the senior physicians mentioned that it was important for the 'good doctor' to know how to establish rapport with patients or to have knowledge about the doctor-patient relationship" (Milton S. Davis, "Attitudinal and Behavioral Aspects of the Doctor-Patient Relationship as Expressed and Exhibited

by Medical Students and Their Mentors," *Journal of Medical Education*, 43 [1968], 338). *See also* Edwin F. Rosinski, "Professional, Ethical and Intellectual Attitudes of Medical Students," *Journal of Medical Education*, 38 (1963), 1016–1022; and George Psathas, "The Fate of Idealism in Nursing School," *Journal of Health and Social Behavior*, 9 (1968), 52–64.

II THE FIRST OF JULY IN TWO HOSPITALS

1. This figure does not include psychiatric residents, nor some research fellows—physicians who have completed their internships and usually some resident training, and who are working on special research projects.

2. "In comparison with the previous year, the overall average of $4,322 is an increase of $525 annually. The average salary in affiliated hospitals was $4,139, an increase of $561, while the average in non-affiliated hospitals was $4,521, an increase of $450 per year" (American Medical Association, *Directory of Approved Internships and Residencies* [1967–68], p. 7). The amount of stipend and fringe benefits may be more important in those hospitals that pay the largest stipends. "Internship in a major teaching hospital, in contrast with other hospital training, was associated with more parental support. These differences were all significant (CR range from 2.5 to 3.7) except for the 1950 private school graduates. Major support by a spouse or self seemed to have no relation" (Fremont J. Lyden, H. Jack Geiger, and Osler L. Peterson, *The Training of Good Physicians* [Cambridge, Mass.: Harvard University Press, 1968], pp. 147–148).

3. "Although the house officer was an employee of the hospital he often personally identified his interests with the School of Medicine rather than with the hospital . . . If he admitted patients to ward beds when it was not absolutely necessary or when the person did not have teaching value, he might be admonished in unpleasant ways by his colleagues. To admit a turkey (uninteresting patient) scored against one in the medical game. The residents evaluated one another regarding the ease or difficulty with which they admitted patients to the wards. A resident who gained a reputation for admitting too many patients to the ward accommodations was known as a 'sieve.' A resident who was known to be a stern gatekeeper for the hospital was a 'rock.' On some services the resident who admitted the most patients was acclaimed 'the sieve of the year.' A truly 'hard rock' went down into 'the pit' (the Emergency Room) to evaluate each prospective admission very carefully. To be known as 'a sieve' was embarrassing to the resident, but the decisions of 'the rock' were probably more hazardous for the patient" (Raymond S. Duff and August B. Hollingshead, *Sickness and Society* [New York: Harper & Row, 1968], p. 114).

4. Morris Rosenberg, referring to individual values, wrote, "Values are not only determinants of action, but are themselves determined by actions which are patterned on the basis of one's position in society. Both values and choices tend to determine one another, and both tend to change in

the direction of greater mutual consistency, thereby leading to reduction of conflict" (Morris Rosenberg, *Occupations and Values* [Glencoe, Ill.: The Free Press, 1957], p. 24).

Hughes postulates a similar approach to career, "a sort of running adjustment between a man and the various facts of life and his professional world . . . It contains a set of projections of himself into the future, and a set of predictions about the course of events in the medical world itself" (Everett C. Hughes, "The Making of a Physician," in *Men and Their Work* [Glencoe, Ill.: The Free Press, 1958], p. 129). Merton wrote in a similar vein, "The social perception is, rather, a by-product, a derivative, of the structure of human relations" (Robert K. Merton, "The Bearing of Empirical Research on Sociological Theory," in *Social Theory and Social Structure* [Glencoe, Ill.: The Free Press, 1957], p. 108).

See also the discussion of a moral code built up by successive definitions of situations, William I. Thomas, "The Regulation of the Wishes," in Logan Wilson and William L. Kolb, eds., *Sociological Analysis* (New York: Harcourt, Brace & Co., 1949), pp. 185–186. Gregory Bateson has described how the individual simplifies, organizes and generalizes his own view of his environment. He imposes his constructions and meanings onto the objective situation. Acts, objects, people are then considered desirable and good and right, or wrong, or deserving of support, or in need of change, in light of the construction. *See* Gregory Bateson, "Cultural Determinants of Personality," in J. McV. Hunt, ed., *Personality and the Behavior Disorders* (New York: Ronald Press, 1944), II, 714–735. *See also* Talcott Parsons, "Youth in the Context of American Society," in *Social Structure and Personality* (New York: The Free Press of Glencoe, 1964), esp. pp. 156–165.

5. *See* Judith Blake and Kingsley Davis, "Norms, Values, and Sanctions," in Robert E. L. Faris, ed., *Handbook of Modern Sociology* (Chicago: Rand McNally & Co., 1964), esp. pp. 458–461. *See also* Florence Kluckhohn and Fred Strodtbeck, *Variations in Value Orientations* (Evanston, Ill.: Row, Peterson and Co., 1961), chap. I; Thomas, "The Regulation of the Wishes," in *Sociological Analysis*, pp. 185–186.

6. *See* Merton's discussion of the relation between the religious convictions of Puritanism and Pietism and the value commitments of science, where it appears that once value-orientations became established they developed a degree of functional autonomy (*Social Theory and Social Structure*, pp. 574–606).

7. Otto Hintze, "Kalvinismus und Staatsräson in Brandenburg zu Beginn des 17ten Jahrhunderts," *Historische Zeitschrift*, 144 (1931), 232, cited in Reinhard Bendix, *Max Weber: An Intellectual Portrait* (Garden City, New York: Doubleday and Company, 1960), p. 69.

8. *See* Max Weber, "Science as a Vocation," in H. H. Gerth and C. Wright Mills, trans. and eds., *From Max Weber: Essays in Sociology* (New York: Oxford University Press, 1946), pp. 129–156.

See also Weber's statement on values, "The shallowness of our routinized daily existence in the most significant sense . . . consists indeed in the fact that the persons who are caught up in it do not become aware, and above all do not wish to become aware, of this partly psychologically, part pragmatically conditioned motley of irreconcilably antagonistic values. They avoid the choice between 'God and the Devil' and their own ultimate decision as to which of the conflicting values will be dominated by the one, and which by the other. The fruit of the tree of knowledge, which is distasteful to the complacent but which is, nonetheless, inescapable, consists in the insight that every single important activity and ultimately life as a whole, if it is not to be permitted to run on as an event in nature but is instead to be consciously guided, is a series of ultimate decisions through which the soul—as in Plato—chooses its own fate, i.e., the meaning of its activity and existence" (Max Weber, *The Methodology of the Social Sciences*, Edward A. Shils and Henry A. Finch, trans. and eds. [Glencoe, Ill.: The Free Press, 1949], p. 18 and *passim*). In a sense the medical profession has helped create the values and beliefs in the larger society which make the profession possible. *See* Bendix's discussion of status groups and their influence as Weber studied them, Bendix, *Max Weber*, pp. 104–107 and *passim*.

9. Etzioni writes, "The vagueness of ultimate values is surely a prerequisite for their integrative function" (Amitai Etzioni, book review, *American Journal of Sociology*, 66 [1961], 534). Mannheim wrote that values may come to be held "with great tenacity and emotional investment that have self-confirming features" (Karl Mannheim, *Ideology and Utopia* [New York: Harcourt, Brace, & Co., 1949], p. 269).

Numerous others have noted and studied the extent to which some value commitments in a group or organization may come to generate action. Value climate refers to the general network of interlocking factors affecting students' values. *See* Allen H. Barton, *Studying the Effects of College Education* (New Haven: Edward W. Hazen Foundation, 1959), p. 60. Speaking of the possible importance of value climate, John Michael states, "When we consider the top half of the aptitude distribution only, the high school climate has as much impact in shaping its seniors' ability as has family background" (John A. Michael, "High School Climates and Plans for Entering College," *Public Opinion Quarterly*, 25 [Winter 1961], 595).

10. Eliot Freidson claims, that the "professional tradition can be kept quite undefiled in such institutions as medical schools, but it cannot help coming into contact with lay tradition in medical practice" (Eliot Freidson, *Patients' Views of Medical Practice* [New York: Russell Sage Foundation, 1961], p. 197).

11. Morris Janowitz, *The Professional Soldier* (Glencoe, Ill.: The Free Press, 1960), p. 126.

12. Emile Durkheim, "Education: Its Nature and Its Role," in Sherwood D. Fox, trans., *Education and Sociology* (Glencoe, Ill.: The Free Press, 1956), p. 89.

13. Robert K. Merton, "Some Preliminaries to a Sociology of Medical Education," in Robert K. Merton, George G. Reader, and Patricia L. Kendall, eds., *The Student-Physician* (Cambridge Mass.: Harvard University Press, 1957), pp. 6–7.

14. James L. Titchener and Maurice Levine, *Surgery as a Human Experience* (New York: Oxford University Press, 1960), p. xi. For a dramatic statement of one man's reaction to donning a professional cloak, *see* George Bohy, "A Belgian Lawyer's Reflections on His Day's Work," *American Bar Association Journal*, 32 (June 1946), p. 361. Janowitz notes the possible influence of distinctive dress on military solidarity in *The Professional Soldier*, pp. 47, 129–130, and *passim*.

15. Talcott Parsons, "Expressive Symbols and the Social System: The Communication of Affect," in *The Social System* (Glencoe, Ill.: The Free Press, 1951), pp. 384–427.

16. *See* Max Weber, "Science as a Vocation," in *From Max Weber*, esp. p. 138.

17. Charles H. Cooley, *Social Organizations* (Glencoe, Ill.: The Free Press, 1956), p. 321. Bernice T. Eiduson, studying creative scientists, makes a similar point: "The really creative ideas have been likened by Kierkegaard to 'paranoid leaps'—for they are antithetical to everything we know, everything realistic, every way in which we are accustomed to thinking about something. Because such 'crazy' thinking takes one out of the reality sphere, one has to be a fairly well stabilized and integrated person, not to be threatened by thinking in bizarre ways, when controls are at a minimum, and letting one's unconscious take over. One can only think crazily enough to produce something really revolutionary or original when he has some strongly entrenched thinking styles on which he can rely and to which he can come home. Without these, the dangers to personality organization are very great, and so frightening that it would be unlikely that one could let his mind go to fantastic proportions and distortions that are necessary to come up with a unique idea. Stylistic ways of thinking and customary ways of being oriented, become intellectual stabilizers, part of the internal security, very much in the same way that reality does" (Bernice T. Eiduson, *Scientists: Their Psychological World* [New York: Basic Books, Inc., 1962], pp. 124–125).

18. Hughes, *Men and Their Work*, p. 17.

19. *Ibid.*, p. 97.

20. Since 1951, when the National Intern Matching Plan was initiated, the number of interns coming to the hospital through the plan has varied widely. It began with seven filled out of the nine posts offered in 1951, going down to one out of ten offered internships in 1954, and then moving slowly back up to seven filled out of ten in 1957, only to drop off to two out of ten the next three years, and then rise again in 1961 to six filled out of ten. In 1966 the number had dropped back again to two nonforeign interns out of thirteen positions offered.

21. Later, this "Dr. G." volunteered to me that he had decided to go into gynecology three years ago (before he came to Community Hospital) and added, "but if Dr. X wants to think I decided here in his service, that is fine." This not unusual experience in field observation, where at least two individuals selectively perceive a situation, signals desirability of checking out more than one report of "the reason" for an event. The differences in reports of a single event recall the Japanese story, *Rashomon*, in which husband, wife, bandit—each participants in a violent scene—see the scene and their part in it in a very different light. *See* R. Akutagawa, *Rashomon and Other Stories* (New York: Liveright Publishing Corp., 1968).

22. Freidson summarizes results from several studies that have dealt with a permissive atmosphere: "By and large, the evidence . . . is mixed and confusing. In some of the few precise studies of permissive leadership in medical settings . . . negative or ambivalent findings were characteristic. Indeed, some of the evidence implied that the effects of permissiveness could be mischievous, increasing 'communication' it is true, but also increasing mistakes. Furthermore, a study by Lefton and his associates implied that the new horizons opened to low-ranking hospital workers by a democratic ideology can make them less satisfied with their jobs than they were before. And finally, with very few exceptions, these studies have taken place in the United States, where, culturally, there is strong pressure toward levelling the appearance if not the fact of difference in status and the exercise of hierarchial authority; their findings may not apply to other settings where subordination is more traditional and acceptable" (Eliot Freidson, "The Sociology of Medicine," *Current Sociology*, 10–11 [1961–1962], 136). *See also* Mark Lefton, Simon Dinitz, and Benjamin Pasamanick, "Decision-Making in a Mental Hospital: Real, Perceived, and Ideal," *American Sociological Review*, 24 (1959), 822–829.

23. Sir William Osler, "A Way of Life," in William H. Davenport, ed., *The Good Physician* (New York: Macmillan Company, 1962), pp. 142–152.

III TRAVELING DIFFERENT PATHS

1. Among the many discussions of the factors related to selective recruitment and evidence of it, *see* Anne Roe, *The Psychology of Occupations* (New York: John Wiley and Sons, 1956), chap. 21; R. K. Kelsall, "Self-Recruitment in Four Professions," in D. V. Glass, ed., *Social Mobility in Britain* (London: Routledge and Kegan Paul, 1954), pp. 308–320; Morris Rosenberg, *Occupations and Values* (Glencoe, Ill.: The Free Press, 1957), pp. 77–92, 124–128; Edward Gross, "The Career," in *Work and Society* (New York: Thomas Y. Crowell Co., 1958), pp. 143–221.

2. "A natural selection process operates in the academic procession toward and through medical school and it may well be that the survivors are the hardier of the species. However, the route does take its [emotional] toll; studies made over the years place the casualties at from 13 to 50 percent"

(Morton Levitt and Ben Rubenstein, "Medical School Faculty Attitudes toward Applicants and Students with Emotional Problems," *Journal of Medical Education*, 42 [1967], 742). *See also* Howard S. Becker, "Notes on the Concept of Commitment," *American Journal of Sociology*, 66 (1960), 36; and for discussions of the notion of cognitive dissonance, *see* Leon Festinger, Henry W. Riecken, and Stanley Schachter, "When Prophecy Fails," in Eleanor E. Maccoby, Theodore M. Newcomb, and Eugene L. Hartley, eds., *Readings in Social Psychology* (New York: Henry Holt & Co., 1958), pp. 156–163.

3. Oswald Hall, "The Stages of a Medical Career," in E. Gartly Jaco, ed., *Patients, Physicians and Illness* (Glencoe, Ill.: The Free Press, 1958), pp. 289–300.

4. Festinger *et al.*, "When Prophecy Fails," pp. 156–163.

5. Jerome E. Carlin, "Current Research in the Sociology of the Legal Profession," presented at the meetings of the American Sociological Association, August 1962. Other studies of lawyers that provide more evidence of this same selective recruitment include: Jack Ladinsky, "Careers of Lawyers, Law Practice, and Legal Institutions," *American Sociological Review*, 28 (1963), 47–54; Arthur Lewis Wood, "Informal Relations in the Practice of Criminal Law," *American Journal of Sociology*, 62 (1956), 48–55; Dan C. Lortie, "Laymen to Lawmen: Law School, Careers, and Professional Socialization," *Harvard Educational Review*, 29 (1959), 352–369; and Hubert J. O'Gorman, *Lawyers and Matrimonial Cases* (New York: The Free Press of Glencoe, 1963), pp. 43–46.

We have presented figures from our own larger studies of interns and residents, and from the Bureau studies of lawyers. Another study of the medical profession that also shows selective recruitment is William A. Glaser, "Internship Appointments of Medical Students," *Administrative Science Quarterly*, 4 (1959), 337–356.

6. Theresa F. Rogers, "Self-Evaluations of Competence," in "Competence and Careers: A Study of Interns and Residents," unpub. Ph.D. diss., Columbia University, 1969, chap. 4.

7. For analyses of the processes involved, *see* Lewis Coser, *The Functions of Social Conflict* (Glencoe, Ill.: The Free Press, 1956), pp. 114, 119; and Becker, "Notes on the Concept of Commitment," pp. 32–40.

8. Niccolo Machiavelli, *The Prince* (New York: Modern Library, 1940), p. 41.

9. Kurt Lewin, *Resolving Social Conflicts* (New York: Harper and Bros., 1948), p. 199. Of the therapeutic relationship, David Mechanic writes: it is "likely that the greater the investment the patient is required to make, the greater will be his commitment to therapy" (David Mechanic, "Role Expectations and Communication in the Therapist-Patient Relationship," *Journal of Health and Human Behavior*, 2 [1961], 195). See also Festinger *et al.*, "When Prophecy Fails," pp. 156–163; Seymour Martin Lipset, Martin A. Trow, and James S. Coleman, *Union Democracy* (Glencoe, Ill.: The Free

Press, 1956), p. 386; Arnold S. Tannenbaum, "Control Structure and Union Functions," *American Journal of Sociology*, 61 (1956), 536–545; Elliot Aronson and Judson Mills, "The Effect of Severity of Initiation on Liking for a Group," *Journal of Abnormal and Social Psychology*, 59 (1959), 177–181.

10. Thomas G. Webster, "Career Decisions and Professional Self-Images of Medical Students," p. 32, advance working paper for members of the Conference on Psychiatry and Medical Education scheduled for March 6–10, 1967, in Atlanta, Georgia, under the auspices of the American Psychiatric Association and the Association of American Medical Colleges.

11. Robert E. Coker, Jr., Bernard G. Greenberg, and John Kosa, "Authoritarianism and Machiavellianism among Medical Students," *Journal of Medical Education*, 40 (1965), 1075, 1077.

12. "Wispe found that most students learned equally well in both sections, with the poorer students doing better in the teacher-centered classes. However, at the two ends of the personality continuum, the learning of the individual student was related to the interaction between his personality type and the teaching method" (Daniel H. Funkenstein, "Possible Contributions of Psychological Testing of the Nonintellectual Characteristics of Applicants to Medical School," *Journal of Medical Education*, 32, part 2 [1957], 105). *See also* Daniel J. Levinson, "Medical Education and the Theory of Adult Socialization," *Journal of Health and Social Behavior*, 8 (1967), 253–265; Peter V. Lee, *Medical Schools and Changing Times* (Evanston, Ill.: Association of American Medical Colleges, 1962).

13. Richard H. Saunders, Jr., "The University Hospital Internship in 1960," *Journal of Medical Education*, 36 (1961), 574.

14. Fremont J. Lyden, H. Jack Geiger, and Osler L. Peterson, *The Training of Good Physicians* (Cambridge, Mass.: Harvard University Press, 1968), pp. 181, 187.

15. Joshua Fishman, cited in Webster, "Career Decisions," p. 32.

16. Levine and Sussmann's study of fraternity pledging notes, "The better he feels he fits the picture, the more often he enters into competition for membership" (Gene Norman Levine and Leila A. Sussmann, "Social Class and Sociability in Fraternity Pledging," *American Journal of Sociology*, 65 [1960], 394).

17. This is not surprising. In a study of school boards, one team of sociologists found more consensus on role definition among superintendents who had undergone similar training programs than among elected members who represent diverse training. *See* Neal Gross, Ward S. Mason, and Alexander W. McEachern, *Explorations in Role Analysis* (New York: John Wiley and Sons, 1958), pp. 146–148. Inkeles states, "since it seems likely that personalities are not randomly recruited to statuses, the effects of the modal personality patterns in any given group of status incumbents may be a massive influence on the quality of role performance in the group" (Alex Inkeles, "Personality and Social Structure," in Robert K. Merton, Leonard

Broom, and Leonard S. Cottrell, Jr., eds., *Sociology Today* [New York: Basic Books, 1959], pp. 266–267).

18. Fleisher compared productivity of groups of medical students and found that groups in which members had shared values were the more productive. *See* Daniel S. Fleisher, "Composition of Small Learning Groups in Medical Education," *Journal of Medical Education*, 43 (1968), 349–355.

19. Chester I. Barnard, *The Functions of the Executive* (Cambridge, Mass.: Harvard University Press, 1956), p. 148.

20. As Hyman observed, "it would certainly seem reasonable that the length of our membership [in a group] would indicate something of our sense of identification or about the degree to which we have internalized its norms" (Herbert Hyman, "Reflections on Reference Groups," *Public Opinion Quarterly*, 24 [1960], 396). Gusfield suggests that it is fruitful to look at how long a person has worked for a given organization as well as how long he has followed on occupation. *See* Joseph R. Gusfield, "Occupational Roles and Forms of Enterprise," *American Journal of Sociology*, 66 (1961), 574. Blau, in studying workers in a government agency, found that "workers with less than three years of experience were less capable of discriminating between various types of supervision than experienced oldtimers" (Peter M. Blau, "Patterns of Deviation in Work Groups," *Sociometry*, 23 [1960], 259).

21. Osler L. Peterson, Leon P. Andrews, Robert S. Spain, and Bernard G. Greenberg, "An Analytical Study of North Carolina General Practice, 1953–1954," *Journal of Medical Education*, 31, part 2 (1956), 67.

Studies of alumni from colleges also suggest the importance of the variable, duration of influence. Newcomb's panel study of attitudes in a small Eastern college found that "those who had spent most time in college not only changed their attitudes most during those years but also maintained their changed attitudes more persistently after leaving college" (Theodore M. Newcomb, *Social Psychology* [New York: Dryden Press, 1950], p. 206). Jacob also reports from his study that "students tended to shed divergent attitudes which they may have brought with them as they became 'seniorized' " (Philip Jacob, *Changing Values in College* [New York: Harper & Bros., 1957], p. 40). Barton writes that a "comparison of different groups at different stages of exposure to college does not, of course, tell us how much of the difference is due to selective dropping out of college by those who deviate . . . and how much represents actual change in attitudes" (Allen H. Barton, *Studying the Effects of College Education: A Methodological Examination of Changing Values in College* [New Haven, Conn.: Edward W. Hazen Foundation, 1959], p. 57). But the ultimate impact of selective recruitment is likely to be exerted regardless of how much is due to selection and how much is due to group reinforcement.

22. Reported in Patricia L. Kendall, "Medical Education as a Social Process," p. 13, paper presented at the Annual Meeting of the American Sociological Association, New York, August 1960.

23. Wheeler describes the effect of expectation for stay in one organization—a prison. *See* Stanton Wheeler, "Socialization in Correctional Communities," *American Sociological Review,* 26 (1961), 697–712.

24. *Ibid,* pp. 698–699, 706.

25. George C. Homans, *The Human Group* (New York: Harcourt, Brace, and Co., 1950), p. 306.

26. For a discussion of this phenomenon in other organizations, *see* Bernard Levenson, 'Bureaucratic Succession," in Amitai Etzioni, ed., *Complex Organizations* (New York: Holt, Rinehart & Winston, 1961), pp. 362–375. French, in his study of a retail organization, observed, "By all measures used . . . these eight men who named friends *more highly placed* than themselves were the most rejected, and rejecting, members of the sales group . . . The effectiveness of the informal controls depended upon the individual's identifying himself with the sales group, but the more he encountered hostility and rejection, the less likely was he to acquire identification" (Cecil L. French, "Correlates of Success in Retail Selling," *American Journal of Sociology,* 66 [1960], 134). Though by no means as competitive as a retail sales group, house-staff members who move toward outside reference individuals may experience small drafts of the same group processes.

27. Careers out of Community Hospital are similar to Oswald Hall's three types of medical careers that he described in a 1949 paper, the "Friendly Career," "Colleague Career," and "Individualistic Career."

In the career of the "friendly physician," satisfaction is derived from personal exchange with patients and with other physicians. He is characterized by intense loyalty to individuals, rather than to institutions. He is not interested in competing with other doctors. He inclines toward cooperation. The "colleague career" includes specialists whose activities are closely related to hospital with house-staff training programs. Such physicians observe their own systems of etiquette in referrals and recommendations. These doctors extend their training through residency and often take part or all of their house-staff training in the community hospital where they hope eventually to practice. Relationships between the physicians and their patients are somewhat circumscribed, formal, organized around appointments, receptionists, nurses, and dignified suites of offices. Prestige in the colleague career relates more closely to social esteem from other physicians and position than to financial success. In this part of the medical system, some of the most promising interns stay in the hospital past residency, waiting their turn to move up as accepted members of the colleague group. The "individualistic medical career" could be pursued somewhat apart from much contact with other physicians. Such a doctor competes for patients and fees and measures success by income and size of practice. This direction tended to keep physicians somewhat suspicious and apart from each other and to stimulate the doctor's rather close attention to the reaction of patients. *See* Oswald Hall, "Types of Medical Careers," *American Journal of Sociology,* 55 (1949), 243–253.

28. Kendall reports: "In the one area in which we have access to reliable data, the filling of internships through the National Intern Matching Plan, the record of the [community] hospital in Community A seems very uneven. In 1957, it offered 8 rotating internships and filled 5 of them . . . In 1958, it offered 12 rotating internships and filled none . . . In 1959, . . . it filled all 10 of the rotating positions offered" (Patricia L. Kendall, *The Relationship between Medical Educators and Medical Practitioners* [Evanston, Ill.: Association of American Medical Colleges, 1965], p. 64). As this report shows, difficulties of community hospitals are related to factors such as superiority of training in the university centers. For the moment, we are considering only the apparent pattern of fluctuation.

Butler and Hage describe the fluctuation of the number of American-trained members in another community hospital. There was only one the second year of the program, then five for the next two years and up to ten, only to be followed by four the next year. The authors cite staff turnover and other reasons. *See* John J. Butler and Jerald T. Hage, "Physician Attitudes toward a Hospital Program in Medical Education," *Journal of Medical Education,* 41 (1966), 913–946. One of the three community hospitals in the town visited for re-evaluation showed marked fluctuation. American-trained interns in the program followed this sequence: 19, 8, 14, 10, 10, 2, 8, 2.

29. For a discussion of size influence on friendship patterns, see Lipset *et al., Union Democracy,* pp. 161, 171–175, and *passim.* What happens within the University Hospital special service seems relevant to the University Hospital house-staff member in a way that recalls the degree of relevancy of union policies for some members of the Typographer's Union. Lipset *et al.* suggest this kind of relevancy may offer a decisive factor in the influence of friendship choice (*ibid.,* p. 96).

Hollingshead discusses the factor of similarity of background in friendship formation. *See* August B. Hollingshead, *Elmtown's Youth* (New York: John Wiley & Sons, 1949), pp. 163–242. Studies in mate selection point to the same factor at work. *See,* for example, Robert F. Winch, *Mate Selection* (New York: Harper & Bros., 1958).

30. Kendall, "Medical Education as a Social Process," p. 11. The impact of social structure on friendship formation is often overlooked, although numerous studies over the past three decades have demonstrated it repeatedly. For example, Merton found that people in a housing project *accounted* for their friendship choice wholly in terms of shared interests and personality compatibility. But statistical analysis of spatial distributions of friendship choices indicated the influence of residential propinquity. *See* Robert K. Merton, "The Social Psychology of Housing," in Wayne Dennis, ed., *Current Trends in Social Psychology* (Pittsburgh: University of Pittsburgh Press, 1948), pp. 163–217. *See also* Homans, *The Human Group,* p.

135 and *passim;* Leon Festinger, Stanley Schachter, and Kurt Back, *Social Pressure in Informal Groups* (New York: Harper & Bros., 1950); Reed M. Powell, "Sociometric Analysis of Informal Groups: Their Structure and Function in Two Contrasting Communities," *Sociometry,* 15 (1952), 367–399; John T. Gullahorn, "Distance and Friendship as Factors in the Cross Interaction Matrix," *Sociometry,* 15 (1952), 123–134. The interaction forced on individuals by their social structure could have an opposite effect from adjustment and friendship. It can make for tension, withdrawal, and the sharpening of boundaries between groups. *See* Leo Kuper, "Blueprint for Living Together," in *Living in Towns* (London: Cresset, 1953), p. 93.

31. *See* Paul F. Lazarsfeld and Robert K. Merton, "Friendship as Social Process: A Substantive and Methodological Analysis," in Monroe Berger, Theodore Abel, and Charles H. Page, eds., *Freedom and Control in Modern Society* (New York: D. Van Nostrand Co., 1954), p. 36.

32. *See* Levenson, "Bureaucratic Succession," pp. 362–375; Robert H. Guest, "Managerial Succession in Complex Organizations," *American Journal of Sociology,* 68 (1962), 47–54; and Alvin Gouldner, "Comment," on Guest, *American Journal of Sociology,* 68 (1962), 54–56.

IV SOCIAL NETWORKS

1. Community size is one of the variables I did not explore early in this study. It is likely that some of the factors we attribute to overlapping commitments between hospital and community are closely related to the fact that this is a relatively small town. Certainly some of the comments of Community Hospital people about interest in the hospital are influenced by community size. For example, the director of nursing at Community Hospital said the local press reported even minor additions to hospital facilities, and suggested community interest in its hospital results in involvement of the individual professional with community expectations. "There are all sorts of lines that cross back and forth."

2. The chances for informal arrangements and for rather wide use of volunteers are probably best in the relatively small hospital in those suburbs where the union poses less threat to the use of volunteers.

3. A study of fourteen medical schools found that even when income level is held constant, marriage rate is a school characteristic, as is the expectation to go into general practice. *See* Louise Ann Johnson, "The Variety in Value Structure of Medical Schools," unpub. Ph.D. diss., Columbia University, 1965, chap. 5, pp. 23, 26.

4. Zetterberg observes that "Increases in outside relations, overlapping memberships, and/or mobility tend to bring an increase in the consensus of communications" (Hans L. Zetterberg, *Social Theory and Social Practice* [New York: Bedminster Press, 1962], p. 83).

5. This may also have undesirable consequences. For example, the community's definitions about priorities for allocating funds may favor patient

comforts or hospital decorations over hiring a full-time member of the teaching staff. *See* Philip Selznick, "Foundations of the Theory of Organization," *American Sociological Review,* 13 (1948), 25–35. *See also* the discussion of processes of organizations and their environments striking an equilibrium in S. N. Eisenstadt, "Bureaucracy, Bureaucratization, and Debureaucratization," in Amitai Etzioni, ed., *Complex Organizations* (New York: Holt, Rinehart, & Winston, 1961), pp. 268–277. And *see* James D. Thompson and William J. McEwen, "Organizational Goals and Environment: Goal Setting as an Interaction Process," *American Sociological Review,* 23 (1958), 23–31.

6. Blankeship and Elling suggest that the hospital may do better in gaining financial support through close personal connections with the power structure of a community, but it loses flexibility. The tail may begin to wag the dog. *See* L. Vaughn Blankeship and Ray H. Elling, "Organizational Support and Community Power Structure: The Hospital," *Journal of Health and Human Behavior,* 3 (1962), 257–269. *See also* Stanley H. Udy, Jr., "Administrative Rationality, Social Setting, and Organizational Development," *American Journal of Sociology,* 68 (1962), 299–308; Burton R. Clark, "Organizational Adaptation and Precarious Values," in Amitai Etzioni, ed., *Complex Organizations* (New York: Holt, Rinehart & Winston, 1961), pp. 159–167. Hanson in a study of hospital administrators, board members, and community leaders found patterned differences in role expectations of administrators and board members that relate to the other positions they held. *See* Robert C. Hanson, "The Systematic Linkage Hypothesis and Role Consensus Patterns in Hospital-Community Relations," *American Sociological Review,* 27 (1962), 304–313.

7. "The very nature of the teaching hospital affords many, many opportunities for informal education" (Alan C. Green, "Educational Facilities in the Hospital for Teaching," *Annals of the New York Academy of Sciences,* 128 [1965], 663).

8. The information about interns and residents at Community Hospital that I gained from people in administration at the hospital, some of whom lived on the grounds with house-staff members, was similar in some respects to information gained from managers about tenants in Merton's housing study. *See* Robert K. Merton, "Selected Problems of Field Work in the Planned Community," *American Sociological Review,* 12 (1947), 304–312.

9. Interns' estimates of the average number of hours they worked at house-staff duties in University Hospital ran from 80 to 140 hours, and averaged 101 hours. Since a week has only 168 hours, these estimates seem high. They may represent understandable tendencies to recall recent "hectic" weeks as an average. In the nationwide survey, 8 percent of the respondents in the large affiliated hospitals reported they were on duty (on call) 136 hours or more in an average week. Only 3 percent of the respondents in the small nonaffiliated hospitals reported such high figures for their "average week."

Interns at Community Hospital reported an average work week of from 60 to 90 hours; their average estimates fell at 71 hours. At University Hospital interns gave estimates ranging from 70 to 115 hours of work per week. One American-trained resident at Community Hospital reported he worked 48 hours a week. *See* Robert K. Merton's discussion of relative deprivation, *Social Theory and Social Structure* (Glencoe, Ill.: The Free Press, 1957), pp. 236–241; and *see also* George H. Mead, *Mind, Self and Society* (Chicago: University of Chicago Press, 1934), p. 138.

10. Lazarsfeld and Thielens observed that college teachers, in institutions where working conditions were objectively good, did not express greater satisfaction with working conditions than their less advantaged colleagues when they evaluated their own colleges. Relative to high expectations or high standards, ratings were low. In University Hospital, interns seem to hold "great expectations" for teachers being "up-to-date," and because of these high expectations they judge attendings harshly. *See* Paul F. Lazarsfeld and Wagner Thielens, Jr., *The Academic Mind* (Glencoe, Ill.: The Free Press, 1958), pp. 25–26.

11. The Cain and Bowen survey reports an increasingly large percentage of house-staff members looking forward to a full-time medical school appointment, and to combination of practice with teaching or research. *See* John Z. Bowers, "Fundamental Purposes of Formal Education beyond Medical School," *Journal of the American Medical Association,* 181 (1962), 387.

A sociological abstraction, the "reference group," points to the sometimes slighted fact that people can measure themselves by using comparisons with people around them, or they can refer to some group or social category beyond and outside their present social position. *See* the following chapters in Herbert H. Hyman and Eleanor Singer, eds., *Readings in Reference Group Theory and Research* (New York: The Free Press of Glencoe, 1968); Robert K. Merton and Alice Kitt Rossi, "Contributions to the Theory of Reference Group Behavior," pp. 28–68; Herbert H. Hyman, "The Psychology of Status," pp. 147–165; Theodore M. Newcomb, "Attitude Development as a Function of Reference Groups: The Bennington Study," pp. 374–386. *See also* Ralph H. Turner, "Reference Groups of Future-Oriented Men," *Social Forces,* 34 (1955), 130–136, and Ralph H. Turner, "Role-Taking, Role Standpoint, and Reference-Group Behavior," *American Journal of Sociology,* 61 (1956), 316–328.

12. Bryan R. Wilson, "The Teacher's Role: A Sociological Analysis," *British Journal of Sociology,* 13 (March 1962), 16. One of the many indicators of increasing emphasis on cumulative scientific efforts in medicine in this country is offered in the report of a consulting engineer to the New York Academy of Medicine in 1958: "of the volumes stored and the volumes used in medical libraries about two-thirds were journals . . . the number of these journals had increased 300 percent in 30 years" (Frederic C. Wood,

"Medical Library Cooperation in New York City," *Bulletin of the New York Academy of Medicine,* 34 [1958], 551).

13. "The expansion of the research establishment in clinical departments and the participation of teacher-investigators in clinical teaching have changed the teaching environment from one based on authority to one that is dedicated to inquiry" (Robert H. Ebert, "Medical Education," *American Review of Respiratory Diseases,* 92 [1965], 554).

14. Herbert A. Simon, *Administrative Behavior: A Study of Decision-Making Processes in Administrative Organizations* (New York: Macmillan Company, 1960), pp. 138–139.

15. A number of studies point to the function of centrality of communication of information for solving a group task. *See* Alex Bavelas, "Communication Patterns in Task-Oriented Groups," in Daniel Lerner and Harold D. Lasswell, eds., *The Policy Sciences* (Stanford: Stanford University Press, 1951), pp. 193–202, and Simon, *Administrative Behavior,* p. 139 and *passim*.

See also James D. Thompson, "Authority and Power in 'Identical' Organization," *American Journal of Sociology,* 62 (1956), 290–301. McCleery suggests the importance of "communication patterns as a basis for system of authority and power" (Richard H. McCleery, "Policy Change in Prison Management," in Amitai Etzioni, ed., *Complex Organizations* [New York: Holt, Rinehart and Winston, 1961], p. 376). Edwin Blakelock notes that "the informal structure of organizations is in part determined by passive contacts between individuals" ("A New Look at the New Leisure," *Administrative Science Quarterly,* 4 [1960], 467).

16. Lazarsfeld and Thielens, *The Academic Mind,* pp. 25–26.

17. Several reports of small-group experiments suggest a tendency for individuals to agree when they are faced with a unanimous judgment of others. This tendency to concur seems to operate whether or not the others are objectively right. *See* S. E. Asch, "Studies in the Principles of Judgments and Attitudes: II. Determination of Judgments by Group and by Ego Standards," *Journal of Social Psychology,* 12 (1940), 433–465; Muzafer Sherif, "Group Influences upon the Formation of Norms and Attitudes," in Eleanor E. Maccoby, Theodore M. Newcomb, and Eugene L. Hartley, eds., *Readings in Social Psychology* (New York: Henry Holt & Co., 1958), pp. 219–232; Robert F. Bales, "Small-Group Theory and Research," in Robert K. Merton, Leonard Broom, and Leonard S. Cottrell, Jr., eds., *Sociology Today* (New York: Basic Books, 1959), pp. 293–305.

18. Merton, *Social Theory,* p. 403.

19. Theodore Caplow and Reece J. McGee, *The Academic Marketplace* (New York: Basic Books, 1958), p. 107.

20. Ronald G. Corwin, "Role Conceptions and Career Aspirations: A Study of Identity in Nursing," *Sociological Quarterly,* 2 (1961), 69–86.

21. Merton, *Social Theory,* p. 402. *See* Patricia L. Kendall's excellent discussion of some of the bases for different orientations of practitioners

and professors, the locals and the cosmopolitans of medicine. Kendall's report is based on interviews from eight communities in the nation, and it is filled with useful material from both cosmopolitans and locals. Kendall discusses some elements in structure that may give rise to different orientations much more thoroughly than I am attempting here. See Patricia L. Kendall, *The Relationship Between Medical Educators and Medical Practitioners* (Evanston, Ill.: Association of Medical Colleges, 1965).

22. Kendall, *Medical Educators and Medical Practitioners*, pp. 97, 98.

V FROM STUDENT TO PHYSICIAN

1. Mary Jean Huntington, "The Development of a Professional Self-Image," in Robert K. Merton, George G. Reader, and Patricia L. Kendall, eds., *The Student-Physician* (Cambridge, Mass.: Harvard University Press, 1957), p. 187. *See also* Charles H. Cooley, *Human Nature and the Social Order* (Glencoe, Ill.: The Free Press, 1956), esp. pp. 183–185; George Herbert Mead, *Mind, Self, and Society* (Chicago: University of Chicago Press, 1934), pp. 138–139; Rose Laub Coser, "Alienation and the Social Structure," in Eliot Freidson, ed., *The Hospital in Modern Society* (New York: The Free Press of Glencoe, 1963), pp. 231–265; Howard S. Becker, Blanche Geer, Everett C. Hughes, and Anselm L. Strauss, *Boys in White* (Chicago: University of Chicago Press, 1961), pp. 316–317.

2. Melvin Prince found a similar pattern in the nationwide study where more than four fifths of the sample of interns and residents stated that they would choose the same internship if they had it to do over. *See* Melvin Prince, "The March toward Doctorship: A Study of the Transition from Medical Student to Intern," Ph.D. diss., Columbia University, 1962.

3. This orientation is what Oswald Hall identified as "colleague career." *See* Oswald Hall, "Types of Medical Careers," *American Journal of Sociology*, 55 (1949), 243–253.

From the sociological perspective, peers become the reference group for physicians who are primarily oriented to research and teaching. *See* the following chapters in Herbert H. Hyman and Eleanor Singer, eds., *Readings in Reference Group Theory and Research* (New York: The Free Press, 1968): Robert K. Merton and Alice Kitt Rossi, "Contributions to the Theory of Reference Group Behavior," pp. 28–68; and Theodore M. Newcomb, "Attitude Development as a Function of Reference Groups: The Bennington Study," pp. 374–386. And *see also* Herbert H. Hyman, "Reflections on Reference Groups," *Public Opinion Quarterly*, 24 (1960), 383–396; Ralph H. Turner, "Reference Groups of Future-Oriented Men," *Social Forces*, 34 (1955), 130–136. Ralph H. Turner, "Role-Taking, Role Standpoint, and Reference-Group Behavior," *American Journal of Sociology*, 61 (1956), 316–328.

4. Charlotte F. Muller, "The Study of Prescribing as a Technic of Ex-

amining a Medical Care System," *American Journal of Public Health,* 57 (1967), 2120.

5. For studies that point to the particularly advantaged position in which a person has regular access to relevant information for solving a group task, *see* Alex Bavelas, "Communication Patterns in Task-Oriented Groups," in Daniel Lerner and Harold D. Lasswell, eds., *The Policy Sciences* (Stanford: Stanford University Press, 1951), pp. 193–202; and James D. Thompson, "Authority and Power in 'Identical' Organizations," *American Journal of Sociology,* 62 (1956), 290–301. McCleery suggests the importance of "communication patterns as a basis for a system of authority and power" (Richard H. McCleery, "Policy Change in Prison Management," in Amitai Etzioni, ed., *Complex Organizations* [New York: Holt, Rinehart and Winston, 1961], p. 376).

There are still other factors which put nurses at Community Hospital in a position where they have good chances to influence interns. For example, interns sometime moonlight by serving as private duty nurses at night. The director of nurses at Community Hospital seemed to recognize that empathy may develop through performance in the nurse's role. "I think interns who have taken care of the case *as a nurse* will be much more willing, and maybe even eager, to talk over the case with the nurse on the floor than they would be if they only had seen the patient as an intern."

6. University Hospital's turnover rate for graduate nurses is higher than that at Community Hospital (60 percent and 30 percent respectively), though at Community Hospital it is still felt that turnover is "too high." One study of nursing turnover reported the highest turnover in the very small and the very large hospitals. *See* Irwin Deutscher, "A Survey of the Social and Occupational Characteristics of a Metropolitan Nurse Complement," Section 1, Survey Report, Part III, in *A Study of the Registered Nurse in a Metropolitan Community* (Kansas City, Mo.: Community Studies, 1956, Publication 105), p. 91. A 1956 survey of turnover among nursing personnel in general hospitals points up the high turnover rates for nurses generally—higher than for female factory workers. But nursing administrators, supervisors, and head nurses within these hospitals showed much lower turnover rates than did other categories of nurses. *See* Eugene Levine, "Turnover among Nursing Personnel in General Hospitals," *Hospitals,* 31 (September 1957), p. 50–53.

7. Rose Laub Coser, "Evasiveness as a Response to Structural Ambivalence," *Social Science and Medicine,* 1 (1967), 206. One study of nurses in hospitals states, "On the floors, it was the younger nurses who were both hardest to keep and most vigorous in rebuffing any perceived officiousness on the part of the medical staff. The head nurses for the most part were older women who had been trained in a day when the doctor's authority was unquestioned. It was to these older women the doctors turned with their problems" (Temple Burling, Edith M. Lentz, and Robert N. Wilson,

The Give and Take in Hospitals [New York: G. P. Putnam's Sons, 1956], p. 113).

8. Patients, as well as nurses, in teaching hospitals may "put the intern down." Rose Coser quotes one patient, "I found out they're nothing but students with their gadgets in their pockets. To me they look like high school boys" (Rose Laub Coser, *Life in the Ward* [East Lansing, Michigan: Michigan State University Press, 1962], p. 61).

9. Intuitively we sense that life is different depending on the size of the pond in which the frog lives. Size is a variable that has been the subject of numerous theoretical discussions as well as field studies in such various context as high schools and hospitals, airports, and factories. Correlations from these studies have linked size with morale, absentee rates, hierarchy, administrative component, and even acceptance or rejection of rumors. These and many other results are reviewed in Roger G. Barker and Paul V. Gump, *Big School, Small School* (Stanford: Stanford University Press, 1964), pp. 31–35 and *passim*.

See also Howard Baumgartel and Ronald Sobol, "Background and Organizational Factors in Absenteeism," *Personnel Psychology*, 22 (1959), 431–443; and R. W. Revans, "Human Relations, Management and Size," in E. Hugh-Jones, ed., *Human Relations and Modern Management* (Amsterdam: North Holland Publishing Co., 1958), pp. 177–220.

For discussions of the relationship between size (moral density) and division of labor, *see* Emile Durkheim, *The Division of Labor in Society*, trans. George Simpson (Glencoe, Ill.: The Free Press, 1933); Ferdinand Toennies, *Fundamental Concepts of Sociology*, trans. C. P. Loomis (New York: American Book Co., 1940); Robert Redfield, "The Folk Society," in Logan Wilson and William L. Kolb, eds., *Sociological Analysis* (New York: Harcourt, Brace & Co., 1949), pp. 349–366.

As Merton observed, "At least since the time of Spencer, it has been noted that there is a distinct tendency for growth to go hand in hand with increasing differentiation" (Robert K. Merton, *Social Theory and Social Structure* [Glencoe, Ill.: The Free Press, 1957], p. 315). But with organizations the matter is much more complex. At some point in size, bigness transforms the structure into a new form. Mason Haire explored the relation between size, shape and function of organizations and suggested a biological model. A dog miraculously enlarged to the size of an elephant would have to have elephant legs to support him. The proportions of the infant must change before he grows to the size of a man. As the organization expands, its internal shape must change. Additional functions of coordination, control and communication must be provided and supported by the same kind of force that previously supported an organization without these things. If the relation were linear, there would be no problem. However, in the organization as in the organism, the proportion of skeleton needed to support the mass grows faster than the mass itself and puts a limit on size as a function of the environmental forces playing on it. *See* Mason Haire, "Biological

Models and Empirical Histories of the Growth of Organizations," in Amitai Etzioni and Eva Etzioni, eds., *Social Change* (New York: Basic Books, 1964), pp. 362–375.

10. Morris Zelditch, Jr., and Terence K. Hopkins rightly observe, "Large size, in our view, is not in itself a critical characteristic of organizations. Rather, what appears to be important here is complexity, which is often indicated by size but is quite distinct from it" ("Laboratory Experiments with Organization," in Etzioni, *Complex Organizations*, p. 470). The primary goals and orientation of an organization seem to enlarge or diminish the effect of size. As we have noted, the environment outside the organization also can play a part in contributing to bureaucratic development. Terrien and Mills, in their empirical study of the effect of size on otherwise similar organizations found that the *proportion* of the administrative component increased with increase in size of organizations. *See* Frederic W. Terrien and Donald L. Mills, "The Effect of Changing Size upon the Internal Structure of Organizations," *American Sociological Review*, 20 (1955), 11–13. Anderson and Warkov challenged the Terrien and Mills findings with their results from their sample of forty-nine Veterans Hospitals. *See* Theodore R. Anderson and Seymour Warkov, "Organizational Size and Functional Complexity: A Study of Administration in Hospitals," *American Sociological Review*, 26 (1961), 23–28. They noted that school districts, which Terrien and Mills had studied, and Veterans Hospitals may differ in the extent to which they may be subject to *centralized* authority. Some administrative increase in Veterans Hospitals could be absorbed by offices outside the hospitals. There could also be administrative increase hidden in the proportion of *time* nonadministrative people in hospitals, for example, nurses and interns, may be devoting to administrative matters, and more bureaucratic forms of communication in the larger hospitals. In addition, the extent of specialization induced by factors other than size, for example, concentration on research, seems to operate to increase more formal patterns of communication.

11. These are by no means all the attributes of that complex enterprise, bureaucracy, which have been pointed out by students of organizations. We have simply pulled out some which appear to make a difference in the experience of house-staff members. For a survey of some of the different writings on bureaucracy, *see* Richard H. Hall, "The Concept of Bureaucracy: An Empirical Assessment," *American Journal of Sociology*, 69 (1963), 32–40; Peter M. Blau and W. Richard Scott, *Formal Organizations* (San Francisco: Chandler Publishing Co., 1962), pp. 42–58; and Merton, *Social Theory*, pp. 310–326. And *see* Weber's discussion of bureaucracy as an ideal type: "Bureaucracy," in H. H. Gerth and C. Wright Mills, trans. and eds., *From Max Weber: Essays in Sociology* (New York: Oxford University Press, 1946), pp. 196–244.

12. Mary Goss, studying physicians in "our" University Hospital's out-patient clinic, found that "Apparently, following administrative regulations

was not very important to physicians when the regulations conflicted with the professional task of taking care of patients whose needs they evaluated as more pressing. Consequently they felt free to disregard administrative requests on occasions when conflicts arose" (Mary E. Weber Goss, "Physicians in Bureaucracy: A Case Study of Professional Pressures on Organizational Roles," unpub. Ph.D. diss., Columbia University, 1959, p. 69). Yet this study also found some correlation between the amount of administrative responsibility the physician had (more as he moved up the hierarchy) and his accepting attitude toward paper work.

13. Mark Lefton, Simon Dinitz, and Benjamin Pasamanick, "Decision-Making in a Mental Hospital: Real, Perceived, and Ideal," *American Sociological Review*, 24 (1959), 828–829.

14. Lipset, Trow, and Coleman found that "in large shops men could form politically homogeneous sub-groups and insulate themselves from the dominant political climate in the shop [of the International Typographical Union], while such insulation was impossible in the smaller shops" (Seymour Martin Lipset, Martin A. Trow, and James S. Coleman, *Union Democracy* [Glencoe, Ill.: The Free Press, 1956], p. 340). In a similar way, and with additional factors supporting the direction, the specialty group in the larger hospital can somewhat insulate itself from some "outsiders" in the hospital.

15. To use David Lockwood's term, the hospital structure determines which people will be in positions of "unavoidable relationships." As Lockwood shows, these "unavoidable relationships" can influence the direction of worker's identification and sympathies. *See* David Lockwood, *The Blackcoated Worker* (London: George Allen & Unwin, Ltd., 1958). And *see* Merton, *Social Theory*, pp. 368–380.

16. However, with the clear rank the surgical group also presents close informality and lack of bureaucratic rigidity as they come to decisions and work. Rose Coser describes these informal patterns in "Authority and Decision-Making in a Hospital: A Comparative Analysis," *American Sociological Review*, 23 (1958), 60.

17. *See* Allen H. Barton, *Studying the Effects of College Education* (New Haven: Edward W. Hazen Foundation, 1959), pp. 56–59. Characterizations of college situations that seem to predispose students to take the college as a reference group, or to become committed to it and retain identification with it as alumni often draw attention to the notion captured in Merton's group property, "extent of social interaction within the group," along with "degree of engagement of members in the group," and "actual" and "expected duration of membership in the group." *See* Merton, *Social Theory*, pp. 311–317. Rogoff found that colleges where many students presumably lived on campus tended to be the ones where a large proportion of graduates contributed to alumni funds. *See* Natalie Rogoff, *Board Member Colleges: A Comparative Analysis* (New York: Bureau of Applied Social Research of Columbia University, 1957).

18. "Adaptation to West Point: A Study of Some Psychological Factors

Associated with Adjustment at the United States Military Academy" (West Point, New York: United States Military Academy, mimeographed, June 1959).

19. Sanford M. Dornbusch, "The Military Academy as an Assimilating Institution," *Social Forces*, 33 (1955), 316–321.

20. James Gould Cozzens, *Guard of Honor* (New York: Harcourt, Brace & Co., 1948), p. 67.

21. James Bordley, III, "Effect of House Staff Training Programs on Patient Care," *Journal of the American Medical Association*, 173 (1960), 1319.

22. Everett Cherrington Hughes, *Men and Their Work* (Glencoe, Ill.: The Free Press, 1958), p. 36.

23. Howard S. Becker and James W. Carper, "The Development of Identification with an Occupation," *American Journal of Sociology*, 61 (1956), 297.

24. Clark Kerr and Abraham Siegel, "The Interindustry Propensity to Strike: An International Comparison," in Arthur Kornhauser, Robert Dubin, and Arthur M. Ross, eds., *Industrial Conflict* (New York: McGraw-Hill Book Co., 1954), pp. 189–212; Alvin W. Gouldner, *Patterns of Industrial Bureaucracy* (Glencoe, Ill.: The Free Press, 1954), esp. pp. 129–133; Vilhelm Aubert and Oddvar Arner, "On the Social Structure of the Ship," *Acta Sociologica*, 3 (1958), 200–219; Rue Bucher and Anselm Strauss, "Professions in Process," *American Journal of Sociology*, 66 (1961), 325–334.

An example of different work activities that might have implications for patterned differences in attitudes toward some aspects of patient care is offered by the fact that University Hospital surgeons may spend a considerable portion of their time in a surgical amphitheater, working as a team over unconscious patients; the medical interns spend more time as a group with patients who can more often respond to, and make demands for, some interpersonal "contact."

VI THE MEDICAL CHART

1. *See* Richard O'Toole, Maxine R. Cammarn, Richard P. Levy, and Lars H. Rydell, "Computer Handling of Ambulatory Clinic Records," *Journal of the American Medical Association*, 197 (1966), 705–709; Bernard S. Glueck, "The Use of Computers in Patient Care," *Mental Hospitals*, 16 (1965), 117–120; Bernard C. Glueck, Jr., "Automation and Social Change," *Comprehensive Psychiatry*, 8 (1967), 441–449.

2. *See*, for example, Howard E. Freeman and Ozzie G. Simmons, *The Mental Patient Comes Home* (New York: John Wiley & Sons, 1963), p. 25; Bernice T. Eiduson, Principal Project Investigator, "Psychiatric Case History Event System: Transcription Procedures with Lexicons," Reiss-Davis Child Study Center, Los Angeles, 1966, p. 1; Gene Nameche, Mary Waring, and David Ricks, "Early Indicators of Outcome in Schizophrenia."

Journal of Nervous and Mental Disease, 139 (1964), 232; Avedis Donabedian, "Evaluating the Quality of Medical Care," *Milbank Memorial Fund Quarterly,* 44, 3, part 2 (July 1966), 173; Peter E. Trainor and Robert P. Whalen, "Evaluation of Quality of Infant Medical Records," *New York State Journal of Medicine,* 67 (1967), 1912. At the turn of the century Adolph Meyer had urged, "We need less discussion of generalities and more records of well-observed cases—especially records of lifetimes—not merely snatches of picturesque symptoms or transcriptions of their meaning in traditional terms" ("Fundamental Conceptions of Dementia Praecox, *British Medical Journal,* 2 [1906], 757).

3. Alphonse R. Dochez, "President's Address," *Transaction of the American Clinical and Climatological Association,* 54 (1938), xviii–xxvi.

4. Albert F. Wesson, "The Social Structure of a Modern Hospital: An Essay on Institutional Theory," unpub. Ph.D. diss., Yale University, 1951, p. 78.

5. Anna M. Pajala and Stuart A. Brody, "Mistakes in Microfilming," *Medical Record News,* 34 (October 1963), 119. Also *see* George McK. Phillips, "Patient Profile Simplifies Communication," *Hospital & Community Psychiatry,* 17 (1966), 310; Graham Beaumont, David Feigal, Richard M. Magraw, Edward C. DeFoe, and James B. Carey, Jr., "Medical Auditing in a Comprehensive Clinic Program," *Journal of Medical Education,* 42 (1967), 359–367; Sister M. Vivian Arts and Sister M. Patrick Klauck, "Utilization Review in Action," *Hospital Progress,* 47 (December 1966), 65–72; Lawrence L. Weed, "Medical Records that Guide and Teach," *New England Journal of Medicine,* 278 (1968), 593–600, 652–657.

6. *See* Theodor D. Sterling and Seymour V. Pollack, *Computers and the Life Sciences* (New York: Columbia University Press, 1965), pp. 3, 17; Joseph Jaffe, "Electronic Computers in Psychoanalytic Research," in Jules Masserman, ed., *Violence and War* (New York: Grune & Stratton, 1963), pp. 160–172; Bernard C. Glueck, Jr., and Marvin Reznikoff, "Comparison of Computer-Derived Personality Profile and Projective Psychological Test Findings," *American Journal of Psychiatry,* 121 (1965), 1156–1161.

7. Lewis Mumford's discussion, "Tentacular Bureaucracy," portrays the paper phenomenon with characteristic perspicacity. *See The Culture of Cities* (New York: Harcourt, Brace & Co., 1938), pp. 226–233.

8. "In specific terms little is actually done to audit the physician or the hospital on routine practices and to evaluate the scientific quality of medical care and teaching. An audit requires the consistent and organized recording of data. I believe that the hospital record can be the focal point for scientific care and training" (Lawrence L. Weed, "A New Approach to Medical Teaching," *Resident Physician,* 13 [July 1967], 77).

9. Weed, "Medical Records that Guide and Teach," p. 597.

10. "Communications theorists have clearly identified the processes through which an excess of messages produces confusion" (Robert K.

Merton, *Social Theory and Social Structure* [Glencoe, Ill.: The Free Press, 1957], p. 356).

11. A survey of psychiatric wards in five general hospitals found that hospitals with the "most complete training programs" were also those where the highest proportion of physicians "enter the nursing station, make chart entries, etc." *See* Lucy D. Ozarin, "Nursing Stations in Psychiatric Units," *Hospitals*, 31 (October 16, 1957), 74–82.

12. At University Hospital the consistency of pressure toward good chart work should predict that this will be an aspect of the intern's work that will be resistant to deterioration. Carl Backman and his associates suggest, "The greater the number of significant other persons who are perceived to define an aspect of an individual's self-concept congruently, the more resistant to change is that aspect of the self" (Carl W. Backman, Paul F. Secord, and Jerry R. Peirce, "Resistance to Change in the Self-Concept as a Function of Consensus among Significant Others," *Sociometry*, 26 [1963], 104).

13. Robert K. Merton, "Social Conformity, Deviation, and Opportunity Structures: A Comment on the Contributions of Dubin and Cloward," *American Sociological Review*, 24 (1959), 177–189. Richard A. Cloward, "Illegitimate Means, Anomie, and Deviant Behavior," in Lewis A. Coser and Bernard Rosenberg, eds., *Sociological Theory* (New York: Macmillan Company, 1965), pp. 562–582.

14. Leo Tolstoy, "A History of Yesterday" (part of an unfinished work), trans. George L. Kline, *Columbia University Forum*, 2, 3 (Spring 1959), 38.

15. "The rebuke which brings the incipient deviant back into line may further alienate the deviant who is somewhat further advanced" (Albert K. Cohen, "The Study of Social Disorganization and Deviant Behavior," in Robert K. Merton, Leonard Broom, and Leonard S. Cottrell, Jr., eds., *Sociology Today* [New York: Basic Books, 1959], p. 468).

16. Some of the comments of house-staff members at University Hospital recall Blau's observation that an instrumental value may become a terminal value. That is, *the chart* rather than the patient or the treatment progress, for a moment, becomes the focus. Peter M. Blau, *The Dynamics of Bureaucracy* (Chicago: University of Chicago Press, 1955), pp. 7, 43.

17. *Ibid.,* p. 93.

18. Merton, *Social Theory*, pp. 317–318; and Robin M. Williams, Jr., *American Society* (New York: Alfred A. Knopf, 1951), pp. 360–365.

19. Merton, *Social Theory*, pp. 351–352.

20. Karl G. Fenn, "Editorial: Progress Report, Committee for the Study of Hospital Standards in Medicine," *Annals of Internal Medicine,* 49 (1958), 964. The initiation of spot chart-review and related talks about them, which one medical director held with family physicians, resulted in improved medical practice in one hospital. *See* Morris L. Jampol, Robert V. Sager,

and Edwin F. Daily, "Continuing Education in Group Practice," *American Journal of Public Health,* 57 (1967), 1749-1753.

21. Merton, *Social Theory,* 319-323, 374-377.

22. Neal Gross, Ward S. Mason, and Alexander W. McEachern, *Explorations in Role Analysis* (New York: John Wiley & Sons, 1958), pp. 289-318.

23. David Seegal, "Teaching Medical Students to Teach," *Journal of Medical Education,* 39 (1964), 1033.

VII NORMS AND COUNTERNORMS

1. Leonard Broom and Philip Selznick, *Sociology: A Text with Adapted Readings* (New York: Harper & Row, 1955), p. 68. Norms are here considered as process and product, and not primarily from the point of view of their impact on behavior and their relative stability. This perspective on process seems justified in view of the dynamic and changing character of house-staff training. It is a short period, and a process. In addition, medicine is changing, as is the individual hospital. Each year another group of recently graduated medical students seems to evolve new norms in their interaction with the hospital.

Among the spokesmen who stress the need for more attention to the changing aspect of norms, and on the degree to which there may *not* be consensus about norms, *see* the following: Denis H. Wrong, "The Oversocialized Concept of Man in Modern Sociology," in Lewis A. Coser and Bernard Rosenberg, eds., *Sociological Theory* (New York: Macmillan Company, 1965), pp. 112-122; Ralf Dahrendorf, "Out of Utopia: Toward a Reorientation of Sociological Analysis," in Coser and Rosenberg, *Sociological Theory,* pp. 209-227; Robert K. Merton and Elinor Barber, "Sociological Ambivalence," in Edward A. Tiryakian, ed., *Sociological Theory and Sociocultural Change* (New York: The Free Press of Glencoe, 1963), pp. 91-120.

Four propositions can be derived from the concept of norms. First, social prescriptions are best understood in relation to specific positions, or statuses. Second, actual behavior may differ from the norm. Third, behavior will indeed differ from a norm unless there are mechanisms in the social structure that induce conformity to it; that is, people have to be induced, encouraged, and reminded to feel in ways that make them believe they should comply with the norm. Fourth, conformity to specific norms can vary from one social structure to another. This statement of norms and the approach of the chapter follows in its first three points the presentation of Judith Blake and Kingsley Davis, "Norms, Values, and Sanctions," in Robert E. L. Faris, ed., *Handbook of Modern Sociology* (Chicago: Rand McNally & Co., 1964), pp. 456-484.

2. Robert K. Merton, "The Ambivalence of Scientists," *Bulletin of the Johns Hopkins Hospital,* 112 (1963), 78. Merton draws attention to the

function of "prior consensus" in *Social Theory and Social Structure* (Glencoe, Ill.: The Free Press, 1957), p. 382.

3. In 1968 a spate of articles in the *Journal of the American Medical Association* dealt with ethical, legal, and religious issues and dilemmas over priorities. The Board of Trustees of the American Medical Association created a special Committee on Religion and Education in 1963, partly in response to new knowledge that raises questions over criteria for death. *See* the following: Paul S. Rhoads, "Medical Ethics and Morals in a New Age," *Journal of the American Medical Association*, 205 (1968), 517–522; James Z. Appel, "Ethical and Legal Questions Posed by Recent Advances in Medicine," *ibid.*, pp. 513–516; Vincent J. Collins, "Limits of Medical Responsibility in Prolonging Life," *ibid.*, 206 (1968) 389–392; Francis D. Moore, "Medical Responsibility for the Prolongation of Life," *ibid.*, pp. 384–386; Howard P. Lewis, "Machine Medicine and Its Relation to the Fatally Ill," *ibid.*, pp. 387–388. *See also* Henry K. Beecher, "Ethical Problems Created by the Hopelessly Unconscious Patient," *New England Journal of Medicine*, 278 (1968), 1425–1430.

4. Merton and Barber, "Sociological Ambivalence," p. 108.

5. Cited in Maurice B. Strauss, ed., *Familiar Medical Quotations* (Boston: Little, Brown & Co., 1968), p. 142. Renée Fox spells out the function of "training for uncertainty" in medical education in "Training for Uncertainty," in Robert K. Merton, George G. Reader, and Patricia L. Kendall, eds., *The Student-Physician* (Cambridge, Mass.: Harvard University Press, 1957), pp. 207–241.

6. Merton and Barber, "Sociological Ambivalence," p. 108.

7. Dr. Sydney Burwell, quoted by G. W. Pickering, "The Purpose of Medical Education," *British Medical Journal*, 2 (1956), 115.

8. Fox, "Training for Uncertainty," pp. 207–241.

9. Mary E. Weber Goss, "Physicians in Bureaucracy: A Case Study of Professional Pressures on Organizational Roles," unpub. Ph.D. diss., Columbia University, 1959, p. 66.

10. Renée Fox describes debates preceding group decisions in research-oriented hospitals and suggests that the exchange enhanced the ability of the group to cope with their problems by strengthening their conviction that they were right. *See Experiment Perilous* (Glencoe, Ill.: The Free Press, 1959), p. 76. Festinger suggests that the person who is forced to make a decision in an ambiguous situation may use the group both as a security operation and as a validity tester. *See* Leon Festinger, "Informal Social Communication," in Dorwin Cartwright and Alvin Zander, eds., *Group Dynamics* (White Plains, N.Y.: Row, Peterson and Company, 1953), pp. 190–203. In a similar vein, Robert L. Hall wrote about the aircraft commanders he studied: "It seems generally agreed that the convergence of attitudes and behavior so often observed in face-to-face groups is a consequence of the need to 'validate' attitudes by consensus, together with the motivation for acceptance in the group." ("Social Influence on the Aircraft

Commander's Role," *American Sociological Review*, 20 [1955], 292). *See also* Stanley Schachter, "Deviation, Rejection, and Communication," *Journal of Abnormal and Social Psychology*, 46 (1951), 190–207.

11. H. H. Gerth and C. Wright Mills, trans. and eds., *From Max Weber: Essays in Sociology* (New York: Oxford University Press, 1946), p. 138.

12. *See* Lewis A. Coser, "Some Functions of Deviant Behavior and Normative Flexibility," *American Journal of Sociology*, 68 (1962), 172–181. *See also* Robert K. Merton, "Social Conformity, Deviation, and Opportunity-Structures: A Comment on the Contributions of Dubin and Cloward," *American Sociological Review*, 24 (1959), 177–189; and William I. Thomas and Florian Znaniecki, "Three Types of Personality," in Talcott Parsons, Edward Shils, Kasper D. Naegele, and Jesse R. Pitts, eds., *Theories of Society* (Glencoe, Ill.: The Free Press, 1961), II, 934–940.

13. Even without stepping beyond established practices, but simply by moving into a crisis situation where he is not formally assigned, the most well-meaning initiative or innovation toward some socially approved end may sometimes bring—not reward—but punishment in the event of non-success. Note the interesting cases that involve "good samaritan" rulings.

14. Oliver Wendell Holmes, "The Young Practitioner," in William H. Davenport, ed., *The Good Physician* (New York: Macmillan Company, 1962), p. 182.

15. "Patients who are involved in research tend to do quite well with regard to clinical improvement, and this is true even of the control group" (H. A. Rashkis, "Does Clinical Research Interfere with Treatment?" *Archives of General Psychiatry*, 4 [1961], 108).

It is a "well-known fact that about two-thirds of patients seem to improve regardless of the type of psychotherapy they have received. Furthermore, the same improvement figure crops up with methods of treatment which are not labeled as psychotherapy, such as that offered by general practitioners, or CO_2 treament" (Jerome D. Frank, Lester H. Gliedman, Stanley D. Imber, Earl H. Nash, Jr., and Anthony R. Stone, "Why Patients Leave Psychotherapy," *Archives of Neurology and Psychiatry*, 77 [1957], 283). *See also* Anthony R. Stone, Jerome D. Frank, Rudolph Hoehn-Saric, Stanley D. Imber, and Earl H. Nash, "Some Situational Factors Associated with Response to Psychotherapy," *American Journal of Orthopsychiatry*, 35 (1965), 682.

"The therapist's potential influence on patients depends as well on the patient's expectations that the therapy will be helpful" (Ezra Stotland and Arthur L. Kobler, *Life and Death of a Mental Hospital* [Seattle: University of Washington Press, 1965], p. 222).

See also Arthur K. Shapiro, "Factors Contributing to the Placebo Effect," *American Journal of Psychotherapy*, 18, Supplement 1 (1964), 73–88; and Paul Lowinger and Shirley Dobie, "What Makes the Placebo Work?," *Archives of General Psychiatry*, 20 (1969), 84–88.

16. Peter M. Blau, *Bureaucracy in Modern Society* (New York: Random House, 1956), p. 51.

17. *Ibid.,* p. 52.

18. Herbert A. Shepard, "The Value System of a University Research Group," *American Sociological Review,* 19 (1954), 460–461.

19. *See* Merton's discussion of the variable, visibility: "apart from this matter of motivation, the convert may also be peculiarly conformist for want of having had first-hand knowledge of the nuances of allowable and patterned departures from the norms of the group which he has lately joined" (Merton, *Social Theory,* p. 352).

20. Turner, in his study of 120 anthropology students, suggests that when the concept of reference group is applicable, subjects sought to exceed the average performance in their reference groups rather than to equal it. Possibly this is due to the fact that his subjects adopt the *standards* rather than the performance levels of their reference groups. *See* Ralph H. Turner, "Reference Groups of Future-Oriented Men," *Social Forces,* 34 (1955), 130–136.

The physician, Oliver Wendell Holmes, wrote, "The young man knows the rules, but the old man knows the exceptions" (Holmes, "The Young Practitioner," p. 175).

21. Merton and Barber, "Sociological Ambivalence," pp. 113–114.

22. The residents in university hospital environments sometimes express their appreciation for having time or "leisure" to consider different possibilities as they work-up patients. In private, nonteaching hospitals, where more patients pay, there may be more emphasis on getting patients in and out quickly.

23. Renée Fox, in her study of a metabolic research unit in another medical-school hospital, noted that many patients considered that becoming an important research subject was an effective, rewarding and admirable way of coping with their situation. Being a part of the research was a basis for achieving high status in the patient community (Fox, *Experiment Perilous,* pp. 108–109).

Studies on hospitalism suggest that from another perspective effective socialization into some aspects of the patient role can have some unfortunate consequences. *See* Hiram L. Gordon and Clarence Groth, "Mental Patients Wanting to Stay in the Hospital," *Archives of General Psychiatry,* 4 (1961), 124–130; Samuel Nadler, Elwin M. Barrett, Don Miller, Mary Ellen Lea, and James Mosier, "Patients Who Choose to Live in the Hospital," Report from the Social Work and Nursing Service of the VA Hospital, Pittsburgh, Pennsylvania, April 1965; and Leo W. Simmons and Harold G. Wolff, *Social Science in Medicine* (New York: Russell Sage Foundation, 1954), pp. 173–193.

24. Fox, *Experiment Perilous,* p. 122. Rose Coser describes patients who had been several times admitted and took a proprietary attitude toward the

hospital. Patients tended to teach others in ways that supported the norms of doctors and nurses. *See* Rose Laub Coser, *Life in the Ward* (East Lansing, Mich.: Michigan State University Press, 1962), pp. 80–88. In another teaching hospital, it was noted that patients who had difficulty meeting medical demands were considered by other patients as "weak." *See* William W. Schottstaedt, Ruth H. Pinsky, David Mackler, and Steward Wolf, "Prestige and Social Interaction on a Metabolic Ward," *Psychosomatic Medicine*, 21 (1959), 131–141. *See also* Rose Laub Coser, "Some Social Functions of Laughter: A Study of Humor in a Hospital Setting," *Human Relations*, 12 (1959), 171–182.

25. Coser, *Life in the Ward*, pp. 80–88.

26. George G. Reader and Mary E. W. Goss, "Medical Sociology with Particular Reference to the Study of Hospitals," *Transactions of the Fourth World Congress of Sociology*, 2 (1959), 147.

27. Eliot Freidson, *Patients' Views of Medical Practice* (New York: Russell Sage Foundation, 1961), p. 203.

28. *Ibid.*, p. 181.

29. Hubert J. O'Gorman, *Lawyers and Matrimonial Cases* (New York: The Free Press of Glencoe, 1963), p. 58.

30. The lower SES patients do of course present other problems of patient management. For example, in one university hospital study of 178 elderly patients in a clinic, it was found that only two fifths of those who did not complete high school made no errors in taking their medications. *See* Doris Schwartz, Mamie Wang, Leonard Zeitz, and Mary E. Weber Goss, "Medication Errors Made by Elderly, Chronically Ill Patients," *American Journal of Public Health*, 52 (1962), 2018–2029.

31. Charles H. Cooley, *Social Organization* (Glencoe, Ill.: The Free Press, 1956), p. 244.

32. The process of creation of norms and agreements I am suggesting is something like that described by Albert Cohen. One member makes a suggestion, another encourages the direction with an act or comment, someone else confirms the direction, so that something new is built on successive definitions of the situation. *See* Albert K. Cohen, *Delinquent Boys* (Glencoe, Ill.: The Free Press, 1955). *See also* William I. Thomas, "The Four Wishes and the Definition of the Situation," in Parsons *et al.*, *Theories of Society*, II, pp. 741–744; William I. Thomas, "The Regulation of the Wishes," in Logan Wilson and William L. Kolb, eds., *Sociological Analysis* (New York: Harcourt, Brace & Co., 1949), pp. 185–186. Sherif found that experimental groups faced with an ambiguous situation may start out with widely divergent perceptions, but their perceptions gradually converge till they establish their own group norm. *See* Muzafer Sherif and Carolyn W. Sherif, *An Outline of Social Psychology* (New York: Harper & Brothers, 1956), pp. 249–260.

33. As Peter Blau notes, "For . . . exclusion to be a threat that discourages deviant tendencies, the individual must first wish to be included

in the group" (Blau, *Bureaucracy in Modern Society*, p. 55). Over-all, the many advantages the University Hospital intern and resident can gain from being an accepted member of his specialty group suggest he would have much to lose should they disapprove of him. Homans suggests that effectiveness of social control rests in the large number of evils a man brings down upon himself from deviation. "His punishment does not fit the crime, but is altogether out of proportion to it" (George C. Homans, *The Human Group* [New York: Harcourt, Brace & Co., 1950], p. 289).

On the function of multiple sanctions and multiple losses from deviation, *see also* William J. Goode, "Norm Commitment and Conformity to Role-Status Obligations," *American Journal of Sociology*, 66 (1960), 246–258; Chester I. Barnard, *The Functions of the Executive* (Cambridge, Mass.: Harvard University Press, 1956), p. 52. The yearly addition of interns to the specialty group may make its own contribution to conformity. Dittes and Kelley suggest that among individuals who equally value their membership in a group, those who feel least accepted are aware of the possiblity of rejection from the group, conform most to its norms. *See* James E. Dittes and Harold H. Kelley, "Effects of Different Conditions of Acceptance upon Conformity to Group Norms," *Journal of Abnormal and Social Psychology*, 53 (1956), 100–107.

34. Peter M. Blau, *The Dynamics of Bureaucracy* (Chicago: University of Chicago Press, 1955), pp. 110–115.

35. Everett Hughes has called attention to the extent that all occupational groups strive for, and actually require some protection from too much visibility by "outsiders" who do not understand some problems the work-group faces. This is particularly true of the professions. *See* Everett C. Hughes, "The Study of Occupations," in Robert K. Merton, Leonard Broom, and Leonard S. Cottrell, Jr., eds., *Sociology Today* (New York: Basic Books, 1959), pp. 442–458.

Merton suggests possible functions of limits to outsider-visibility on professional performance. Merton, *Social Theory*, pp. 374–375.

36. Social cohesion does not seem to depend on basic equality of status as Blau claims. *See* Peter M. Blau, "The Dynamics of Bureaucracy," in Amitai Etzioni, ed., *Complex Organizations* (New York: Holt, Rinehart and Winston, 1961), p. 347. There are more ranks and more clearly defined ranks within specialty at University Hospital than at Community Hospital, and yet the University Hospital specialty groups seem more cohesive.

It seems to me that some basic identity of normative interest and some close interaction over common problems is more relevant to cohesiveness than is equality or rank. The fighting group in wartime, for example, may be very cohesive though there are clear rank differences within it.

The work context of the University Hospital learning groups may cast house staff concern for symbols of rank into the future and away from now, as Shepard describes with the research scientists he studied. University Hospital specialty groups produce little ambiguity of status distinctions—

ambiguity that could heighten sensitivity and competitiveness over status symbols with possibly mischievous results against group solidarity. Also, they know they will move up soon after training. *See* Shepard, "The Value System," 456–462.

Tunstall describes another very different work group, but one that is also cut off from outside influence—even more dramatically—and thrown with their superior. These are fishermen who go on twenty-one-day trawling voyages. The author describes their strong loyalties and the impact of their work on their total life. Unlike workers in many other extreme isolated occupations, the fisherman's labor union is neither strong nor militant. Here again, I suggest that a significant variable is the presence of different ranks that might help explain why this occupation group behaves so differently from those in other occupations where men are thrown into close interaction and some danger, for example, the miners. *See* Jeremy Tunstall, *The Fishermen* (London: MacGibbon & Kee, 1962).

37. Work groups somewhat isolated from managements in a plant, for example, seem most likely to create norms—like limitation of output—in opposition to expectations of management. *See* Stanley E. Seashore, *Group Cohesiveness in the Industrial Work Group* (Ann Arbor, Mich.: Institute for Social Research, University of Michigan, 1954), pp. 63–80; and Stanley Schachter, Norris Ellertson, Dorothy McBride, and Doris Gregory, "An Experimental Study of Cohesiveness and Productivity," in Cartwright and Zander, *Group Dynamics,* pp. 401–411.

On the university campus, when fraternity life is essentially isolated from regular or informal interaction with faculty, interaction among peers can lead to norms that interfere with student's academic achievement and scholastic standards. *See* Gene Norman Levine and Leila A. Sussman, "Social Class and Sociability in Fraternity Pledging," *American Journal of Sociology,* 65 (1960), 391–399; R. H. Knapp and H. B. Goodrich, *Origins of American Scientists* (Chicago: University of Chicago Press, 1952); and Jacqueline Pindall Wiseman, "Achievement and Motivation in a College Environment," *Berkeley Journal of Sociology,* 6 (1961), 35–51. Teenagers separated off into their own tight groups can evolve norms that make alarming headlines. *See* Cohen, *Delinquent Boys.*

Medical students who are somewhat cut off from regular interaction with medical faculty can develop patterns and agreement that encourage evasion of some faculty expectations. I am suggesting that the extent and nature of patterned evasions evolved in groups of medical students described by Becker *et al.* is in part a function of the first-year separation of students from medical faculty in the particular school. More research is needed to make this suggestion more than speculation, but patterned evasions could theoretically evolve either in support of, or in subversion of faculty's goals. The direction of patterned evasions, I think, has something to do with whether or not faculty is thrown into frequent and informal interaction with the group of students. *See* Howard S. Becker, Blanche Geer, Everett C.

Hughes, and Anselm L. Strauss, *Boys in White* (Chicago: University of Chicago Press, 1961), pp. 80–91, 107–157, and *passim*.

38. *See* Chester Barnard's discussion of the importance of daily information for decisions that make sense and effective leadership, *The Functions of the Executive*, pp. 185–199.

39. Merton and Barber, "Sociological Ambivalence," p. 112.

40. Max Weber, *The Methodology of the Social Sciences*, Edward A. Shils and Henry A. Finch, trans. and eds. (Glencoe, Ill.: The Free Press, 1949), pp. 23–24.

41. Leland S. McKittrick, "Specialty Practice," in Joseph Garland, ed., *The Physician and His Practice* (Boston: Little, Brown & Co., 1954), p. 67.

42. "Only by strict specialization can the scientific worker become fully conscious, for once and perhaps never again in his lifetime, that he has achieved something that will endure. A really definitive and good accomplishment is today always a specialized accomplishment. And whoever lacks the capacity to put on the blinders, so to speak, and come upon the idea that the fate of his soul depends upon whether or not he makes the correct conjecture at this passage of this manuscript may as well stay away from science" (Gerth and Mills, *From Max Weber*, p. 135).

43. Patricia L. Kendall and Hanan C. Selvin, "Tendencies toward Specialization in Medical Training," in Merton *et al.*, *The Student-Physician*, pp. 153–174.

44. *Ibid.*, p. 156.

45. Lois Pratt, Arthur Seligmann, and George Reader, "Physicians' Views of the Level of Medical Information among Patients," in E. Gartly Jaco, ed., *Patients, Physicians and Illness* (Glencoe, Ill.: The Free Press, 1958), p. 223.

46. *Ibid.*, p. 228.

47. Pellegrino suggests the complexity of consequences arising from different types of training: "It is axiomatic that the best patient care occurs where teaching and research flourish, but something may be gained if it is not assumed that the relationship is absolute" (Edmund D. Pellegrino, "Care of the Patient in the Medical School Setting," *Journal of the American Medical Association*, 173 [1960], 1293).

48. Daniel H. Funkenstein, "A New Breed of Psychiatrist?" *American Journal of Psychiatry*, 124 (1967), 227.

49. Robert H. Ebert, cited in Strauss, *Familiar Medical Quotations*, p. 369.

50. Tuchman suggests the emergency room increasingly "replaces" the family doctor for a large segment of the population. Occasionally, interns or residents complain of families using the emergency room when they "could just as well" wait to see a doctor of their own the next day. *See* Lester E. Tuchman, "Immediate and Long-Range Problems in the Municipal Hospitals of New York City," *Bulletin of the New York Academy of Medicine*, 37 (1961), 537–541.

51. Numerous studies have dealt with some implications of separation of the individual from the outside as he becomes increasingly a part of the hospital world of the sick. *See* Leon Lewis and Rose L. Coser, "The Hazards in Hospitalization," *Hospital Administration*, 5, 3, (Summer 1960), 25–45. *See also* William Caudill, "Applied Anthropology in Medicine," in A. L. Kroeber, ed., *Anthropology Today* (Chicago: University of Chicago Press, 1953), pp. 771–806; H. Warren Dunham and S. Kirson Weinberg, *The Culture of the State Hospital* (Detroit: Wayne State University Press, 1960); Erving Goffman, "The Characteristics of Total Institutions," in Amitai Etzioni, ed., *Complex Organizations* (New York: Holt, Rinehart and Winston, 1961), pp. 312–340; and Esther Lucile Brown, *Newer Dimensions of Patient Care* (New York: Russell Sage Foundation, 1961–1962), part 1.

52. Talcott Parsons wrote, "individuality and creativity are, to a considerable extent, phenomena of the institutionalization of expectations" ("An Outline of the Social System," in Parsons *et al.*, *Theories of Society*, I, 38). Rose Coser, in her comparison of role relationships on a surgical service and on a medical service within one hospital, observed, " 'ritualism' or 'innovation' is largely a function of the specific social structure rather than merely a 'professional' or 'character' trait" (Rose Laub Coser, "Authority and Decision-Making in a Hospital: A Comparative Analysis," *American Sociological Review*, 23 [1958], 63).

VIII PATIENT AND PHYSICIAN

1. In the nationwide survey, nearly half of the respondents in small, nonaffiliated hospitals, but well under one third of the respondents in closely affiliated hospitals, said they *"almost never"* encountered a hostile patient.

2. See David Riesman, "Medical Ethics," in William H. Davenport, ed., *The Good Physician* (New York: Macmillan Company, 1962), pp. 309–313.

3. Zetterberg's observation seems appropriate: "Anything perceived as maintaining the favorable evaluations received by individuals becomes subject to their emotive evaluation" (Hans L. Zetterberg, *Social Theory and Social Practice* [New York: Bedminster Press, 1962], p. 102).

4. Oliver Wendell Holmes, cited in Maurice B. Strauss, ed., *Familiar Medical Quotations* (Boston: Little, Brown & Co., 1968), p. 454.

5. This factor operating in relationships between local practitioners and full-time professors is more completely developed in Patricia L. Kendall, *The Relationship between Medical Educators and Medical Practitioners: Sources of Strain and Occasions for Cooperation* (Evanston, Ill.: Association of American Medical Colleges, 1965).

6. What happens in medicine around the patient-physician relationship is an example of goal displacement. *See* the discussion of goal displacement in a bureaucracy in Robert K. Merton, "Bureaucratic Structure and Person-

ality," in *Social Theory and Social Structure* (Glencoe, Ill.: The Free Press, 1957), pp. 195–206.

7. Kenneth F. Clute, *The General Practitioner: A Study of Medical Education in Ontario and Nova Scotia* (Toronto: University of Toronto Press, 1963), p. 223.

8. Erving Goffman, *The Presentation of Self in Everyday Life* (Garden City, New York: Doubleday & Company, 1959), pp. 17–76.

9. *See* M. Ralph Kaufman, Abraham N. Franzblau, and David Kairys, "The Emotional Impact of Ward Rounds," *Journal of the Mount Sinai Hospital* 23 (1956), 784.

10. Milton S. Davis, "Attitudinal and Behavioral Aspects of the Doctor-Patient Relationship as Expressed and Exhibited by Medical Students and Their Mentors," *Journal of Medical Education,* 43 (1968), 342.

11. Robert F. Loeb, cited in Strauss, *Familiar Medical Quotations,* p. 368.

12. Eliot Freidson, *Patients' Views of Medical Practice* (New York: Russell Sage Foundation, 1961), pp. 152–168.

13. There is some evidence that even among welfare patients, more sophisticated symbols of competence may be used, for example, equipment and bright, modern offices. *See* Daniel Rosenblatt and Edward A. Suchman, "Awareness of Physician's Social Status within an Urban Community," *Journal of Health and Human Behavior,* 7 (1966), 153.

14. Carl A. Moyer, "The Residency Program in a University-Affiliated Hospital: Organization and Administration," *Journal of the American Medical Association,* 161 (1956), 29–32.

15. Seymour Parker observes this phenomenon in "Status Consistency and Stress," *American Sociological Review,* 28 (1963), 132.

16. Milton S. Davis suggests that "one of the basic problems in the relationship between a doctor and a patient is that the expectations that each has for the other are rarely congruent" ("Variations in Patients' Compliance with Doctors' Orders: Analysis of Congruence between Survey Responses and Results of Empirical Investigations," *Journal of Medical Education,* 41 [1966], 1037). Among the important studies of compliance *see* Davis, "Attitudinal and Behavioral Aspects," pp. 337–343; Milton S. Davis, "Predicting Non-Compliant Behavior," *Journal of Health and Social Behavior,* 8 (1967), 265–271; Milton S. Davis, "Variations in Patients' Compliance with Doctors' Advice: An Empirical Analysis of Patterns of Communication," *American Journal of Public Health,* 58 (1968), 274–288; W. J. Johannsen, G. A. Hellmuth, and T. Sorauf, "On Accepting Medical Recommendations: Experiences with Patients in a Cardiac Work Classification Unit," *Archives of Environmental Health,* 12 (1966), 63–69.

17. Robin F. Badgley and Marilyn A. Furnal, "Appointment Breaking in a Pediatric Clinic," *Yale Journal of Biology and Medicine,* 34 (1961), 117–123. John J. Walsh, Jess L. Benton, Jr., Iola G. Arnold, "Why Patients Break Appointments," *Hospital Topics,* 45, 2 (February 1967), 67–72; J.

Philip Ambuel, Jan Cebulla, Norman Watt, and Douglas P. Crowne, "Urgency as a Factor in Clinic Attendance," *American Journal of Diseases in Children,* 108 (1964), 394–398. Robert L. Nolan, Jerome L. Schwartz, and Kenneth Simonian, "Social Class Differences in Utilization of Pediatric Services in a Prepaid Direct Service Medical Care Program," *American Journal of Public Health,* 57 (1967), 34–47.

Among studies that relate to defection from psychotherapy, see the following: Jerome D. Frank, Lester H. Gliedman, Stanley D. Imber, Earl H. Nash, Jr., and Anthony R. Stone, "Why Patients Leave Psychotherapy," *Archives of Neurology and Psychiatry,* 77 (1957), 283–299. Richard L. Cohen and Charles H. Richardson, "A Retrospective Study of Case Attrition in a Child Psychiatry Clinic," presented at the 44th Annual Meeting of the American Orthopsychiatric Association, Washington, D.C., March 1967. Bernice T. Eiduson, "Retreat from Help," *American Journal of Orthopsychiatry,* 37 (1967), 268; Harold Korner, "Abolishing the Waiting List in a Mental Health Center," *American Journal of Psychiatry,* 120 (1964), 1097–1100; O. Eugene Baum and Stanton B. Felzer, "Activity in Initial Interviews with Lower-Class Patients," *Archives of General Psychiatry,* 10 (1964), 345–353; and Joe Yamamoto and Marcia Kraft Goin, "On the Treatment of the Poor," *American Journal of Psychiatry,* 122 (1965), 267–271.

18. "Some studies have demonstrated that the greater the discrepancy between what patients and families expected from the clinic and what the clinic had to offer, the greater the likelihood of attrition" (Cohen and Richardson, "A Retrospective Study of Case Attrition," p. 2).

19. Dr. Ross, discussant in T. S. Danowski, Arthur Krosnick, and Harvey C. Knowles, Jr., eds., "Discussion after Workshop Groups E, F, G, and H," *Juvenile Diabetes: Adjustment and Emotional Problems,* proceedings of a workshop held at Princeton, New Jersey, April 1963, p. 108. In the same proceedings, *see* the following: Leo P. Krall, chairman, "Report of Workshop Group H," p. 101; Edward Wellin, chairman, "Report of Workshop Group C," pp. 63–65; Mabel Ross, chairman, "Report of Workshop Group F," pp. 91–93.

For additional information *see* T. Franklin Williams, Dan A. Martin, Michael D. Hogan, Julia D. Watkins, and E. V. Ellis, "The Clinical Picture of Diabetic Control: Studied in Four Settings," *American Journal of Public Health,* 57 (1967), 441–451; Julia D. Watkins, T. Franklin Williams, Dan A. Martin, Michael D. Hogan, and E. Anderson, "A Study of Diabetic Patients at Home," *ibid.,* pp. 452–459; Henry Dolger and Bernard Seeman, *How to Live with Diabetes* (New York: Pyramid Books, 1958), esp. pp. 129–144; Edwin W. Gates, "Therapy: Teaching of the Patient," in T. S. Danowski, ed., *Diabetes Mellitus: Diagnosis and Treatment* (New York: American Diabetes Association, 1964), pp. 103–107; Donnell D. Etzwiler and Lloyd K. Sines, "Juvenile Diabetes and Its Management: Family, Social, and Academic Implications," *Journal of the American Medical Association,* 181 (1962), 304–308; Joseph M. Worth and Joseph C. Shipp, "Juvenile Diabetes:

The Educational Experience of Diabetic Camp Using Programmed Instruction," *Southern Medical Journal,* 59 (1966), 585–588.

20. *See* George G. Reader and Mary E. W. Goss, "Medical Sociology with Particular Reference to the Study of Hospitals," *Transactions of the Fourth World Congress of Sociology,* 2 (1959), 139–152. Johannsen *et al.* note that "the difficulty in obtaining compliance lies not in the area of communication, but in the psychological readiness of the patient" (Johannsen *et al.,* "On Accepting Medical Recommendations," p. 68). *Also see* Gordon, "Are We Seeing," p. 133; Baum and Felzer, "Activity in Initial Interviews," pp. 345–353; and Kathryn M. Healy, "Does Preoperative Instruction Make a Difference?" *American Journal of Nursing,* 68 (1968), 62–67.

21. Minna Field, *Patients Are People: A Medical-Social Approach to Prolonged Illness,* 3d ed. (New York: Columbia University Press, 1967), p. 39.

22. *See* Hugh A. Storrow, "Social Class and Medical Practice," *Southern Medical Journal,* 56 (1963), 385; Lloyd H. Rogler and August B. Hollingshead, "The Puerto Rican Spiritualist as a Psychiatrist," *American Journal of Sociology,* 67 (1961), 21; Lyle Saunders, *Cultural Difference and Medical Care* (New York: Russell Sage Foundation, 1954), p. 144; Vance Randolph, *Ozark Superstitions* (New York: Dover Publications, 1964), p. 115.

23. Allen D. Spiegel, "Unanswered and Unasked Questions of Hospital Patients," presented at the 94th Annual Meeting of the American Public Health Association, San Francisco, November 1966; and Dorothy T. Linehan, "What Does the Patient Want to Know?" *American Journal of Nursing,* 66 (1966), 1066–1068; John D. Stoeckle, Irving Zola, and Gerald E. Davidson, "On Going to See the Doctor: The Contributions of the Patient to the Decision to Seek Medical Aid," *Journal of Chronic Diseases,* 16 (1963), 975–989; Marc H. Hollender and Leonard A. Stine, "The Medical Patient," in *The Psychology of Medical Practice* (Philadelphia: W. B. Saunders Company, 1958), pp. 35–87.

24. D. F. Preston and F. L. Miller, "The Tuberculosis Outpatient's Defection from Therapy," *American Journal of Medical Sciences,* 247 (1964), 21–24.

25. Herbert S. Caron and Harold P. Roth, "Patients' Cooperation with a Medical Regimen: Difficulties in Identifying the Noncooperator," *Journal of the American Medical Association,* 203 (1968), 922.

26. Davis, "Physiologic, Psychological and Demographic Factors in Patient Compliance with Doctors' Orders," *Medical Care,* 6 (1968), pp. 116, 118, 121; and Davis, "Variations in Patients' Compliance with Doctors' Orders," pp. 1037–1048.

27. Amasa B. Ford, Ralph E. Liske, Robert S. Ort, and John C. Denton, *The Doctor's Perspective: Physicians View Their Patients and Practice* (Cleveland: The Press of Case Western Reserve University, 1967), p. 24.

28. Rose Laub Coser, *Life in the Ward* (East Lansing: Michigan State University Press, 1962), p. 61.

29. Oscar Lewis, *La Vida* (New York: Random House, 1966), p. 265.

30. Ailon Shiloh, "Equalitarian and Hierarchal Patients: An Investigation among Hadassah Hospital Patients," *Medical Care, 3* (April–June 1965), 89.

31. Robert Straus, "Sociological Determinants of Health Beliefs and Behavior," *American Journal of Public Health, 51* (1961), 1550–1551.

32. Hans Popper, "New Curriculum," *Annals of the New York Academy of Sciences, 128* (1965), 553; and Citizens Commission of Graduate Medical Education, *The Graduate Education of Physicians* (Millis Report) (Chicago: American Medical Association, 1966), pp. 43–44.

33. *See* Lawrence S. Kubie, "A School of Psychological Medicine within the Framework of a Medical School and University," *Journal of Medical Education, 39* (1964), 476–480; Wilford W. Spradlin, "Drama as an Adjunct to Teaching Human Behavior," *Journal of Medical Education, 41* (1966), 377–380; Walter J. McNerney, "Comprehensive Personal Health Care Services: A Management Challenge to the Health Professions," *American Journal of Public Health, 57* (1967), 1717–1727; Frank R. Lock, "Preparing the Doctor to Be a Doctor," *American Journal of Obstetrics and Gynecology, 97* (1967), 583–589; W. W. Holland, Jessie Garrad, and A. E. Bennett, "A Clinical Approach to the Teaching of Social Medicine," *Lancet, 1* (1966), 540–542; Jan H. Pfouts and Gordon E. Rader, "Instruction in Interviewing Technique in the Medical School Curriculum: Report of a Trial Program and Some Suggestions," *Journal of Medical Education, 37* (1962), 681–686; and Robert J. Thurnblad and R. Layton McCurdy, "Human Behavior and the Student Physician," *Journal of Medical Education, 42* (1967), 158–162.

34. Warren R. Young, "Rx: For Modern Medicine Some Sympathy Added to Science," *Life* (October 12, 1959), p. 153. There are two assumptions in many current criticisms that I hope I do *not* further by suggesting the possible effects of house-staff commitment to specialization; first, the unproven assumption that the specialist with a relatively narrow focus of expertness is necessarily narrow in other aspects of his life, or blind to other aspects of patient care; second, the nostalgic notion that doctors in the past were uniformly interested in, or knowledgeable about "the total patient." *See* Cecil Woodham-Smith, *Florence Nightingale* (New York: McGraw-Hill Book Co., 1951) for a description of how some patients fared during the middle and late nineteenth century.

35. Dana W. Atchley, "The Science, the Art, and the Heart of Medicine," *Journal of Medical Education, 34,* part 2 (1959), 19.

36. Lester J. Evans, *The Crisis in Medical Education* (Ann Arbor: University of Michigan Press, 1965), pp. 62, 63.

37. M. Ralph Kaufman, Samuel Lehrman, Abraham N. Franzblau, Samuel Tabbat, Leonard Weinroth, and Stanley Friedman, "Psychiatric Findings in Admissions to a Medical Service in a General Hospital," *Journal of the Mount Sinai Hospital, 26* (1959), 160–170; N. Egerton and J. H. Kay, "Psychological Disturbances Associated with Open Heart Surgery," *British*

Journal of Psychiatry, 110 (1964), 433–439; Barney M. Dlin, William Winters, Jr., H. Keith Fischer, and Peter Koch, "Psychological Adaptation to Pacemaker Following Cardiac Arrest," *Psychosomatics,* 7 (1966), 73–80; Jacov Lerner and Pinchas Noy, "Somatic Complaints in Psychiatric Disorders: Social and Cultural Factors," *International Journal of Social Psychiatry,* 14 (1968), 145–150; J. G. Henderson, "Denial and Repression as Factors in Delay of Patients with Cancer Presenting Themselves to the Physician," *Annals of the New York Academy of Sciences,* 125 (1966), 856–864; Bennett L. Rosner, "The Use of Valid Psychological Complaints to Screen, Minimize or Deny Serious Somatic Illness," *Journal of Nervous and Mental Disease,* 143 (1966), 234–238; Mannuccio Mannucci and M. Ralph Kaufman, "The Psychiatric Inpatient Unit in a General Hospital: A Functional Analysis," *American Journal of Psychiatry,* 122 (1966), 1329–1343; and E. I. Burdock, Leah Glass, Anne S. Hardesty, and Yvonne M. Beck, "A Sample Survey of Mental Hospital Patients," *Journal of Clinical Psychology,* 17 (1961), 253–259.

38. M. Ralph Kaufman, "Psychiatry in Medicine: Sibling or Stepchild?" *Maryland State Medical Journal,* 10 (1961), 245; P. Noy, A. Kaplan De-Nour, and R. Moses, "Discrepancy between Expectations and Service in Psychiatric Consultation," *Archives of General Psychiatry,* 14 (1966), 651–657; Eugene B. Piedmont, "Referrals and Reciprocity: Psychiatrists, General Practitioners and Clergymen," *Journal of Health and Social Behavior,* 9 (1968), 33; John E. Schowalter and Albert J. Solnit, "Child Psychiatry Consultation in a General Hospital Emergency Room," *Journal of the American Academy of Child Psychiatry,* 5 (1966), 547; and Felix Deutsch, M. Ralph Kaufman, and Herrman L. Blumgart, "Present Methods of Teaching," *Psychosomatic Medicine,* 2 (1940), 214–215; Thomas R. Kearney, "Psychiatric Consultation in a General Hospital," *British Journal of Psychiatry,* 112 (1966), 1237.

See also John J. Schwab and Judith Brown, "Uses and Abuses of Psychiatric Consultation," *Journal of the American Medical Association,* 205 (1968), 65–68; Z. J. Lipowski, "Review of Consultation Psychiatry and Psychosomatic Medicine," *Psychosomatic Medicine,* 29 (1967), 153–171; John J. Schwab, Roy S. Clemmons, M. J. Valder, and J. D. Raulerson, "Medical Inpatients' Reaction to Psychiatric Consultations," *Journal of Nervous and Mental Disease,* 142 (1966), 215–222; Werner M. Mendal and Philip Solomon, eds., *The Psychiatric Consultation* (New York: Grune & Stratton, 1968), esp. pp. 1–12, 13–17, 26–32, 196–215.

39. But this is changing. "A sign of this is the increased number of psychiatric units in general hospitals [1961]. Relatively few such facilities existed twenty-five years ago. Today there are perhaps six hundred psychiatric departments in such hospitals" (Kaufman, "Psychiatry in Medicine: Sibling or Stepchild?" p. 245).

40. Cited in Henry A. Davidson, "The Image of the Psychiatrist," *American Journal of Psychiatry,* 121 (1964), 331.

41. John G. Bruhn and Oscar A. Parsons, "Medical Student Attitudes

Toward Four Medical Specialties," *Journal of Medical Education,* 39 (1964), 40–49.

42. Cited in Thomas G. Webster, "Career Decisions and Professional Self-Images of Medical Students," advance working paper for members of the Conference on Psychiatry and Medical Education, scheduled for March 6–10, 1967, Atlanta, Georgia, under the auspices of the American Psychiatric Association and the Association of American Medical Colleges, pp. 42–43.

43. H. J. Walton, J. Drewery, and G. M. Carstairs, "Interest of Graduating Medical Students in Social and Emotional Aspects of Illness," *British Medical Journal,* 2 (1963), 588–592.

44. John G. Bruhn and Oscar A. Parsons, "Attitudes Toward Medical Specialties: Two Follow-Up Studies," *Journal of Medical Education,* 40 (1965), 277.

45. John G. Bruhn and Andrea duPlessis, "Wives of Medical Students: Their Attitudes and Adjustments," *Journal of Medical Education,* 41 (1966), 383.

46. Paul Kaufman, "Consultation Services," *International Psychiatry Clinics,* 3, 3 (1966), 128.

47. Sidney L. Werkman, *The Role of Psychiatry in Medical Education* (Cambridge, Mass.: Harvard University Press, 1966), p. 19; Pietro Castelnuovo-Tedesco, "How Much Psychiatry Are Medical Students Really Learning?" *Archives of General Psychiatry,* 16 (1967), 668–675.

Lindsay Beaton discussed some of the reasons that psychiatry often "does not seem to take," in "Psychiatric Necessities in Surgical Education," *American Journal of Surgery,* 110 (1965), 32.

Leo Shatin and Robert P. Nenno write about a psychiatric course: "The most frequent student criticism . . . pertained to excessive diffuseness and lack of structure . . . followed by the criticism . . . that too little substantive content was learned" ("A Behavioral Sciences Teaching Program for First Year Medical Students," *Journal of Medical Education,* 38 [1963], 846).

48. Emily Mumford, "Teacher Response to School Mental Health Programs," *American Journal of Psychiatry,* 125 (1968), 75–81. Russell Monroe reports three patterns within the medical student population he studied. *See* Russell R. Monroe, "Techniques for Evaluating the Effectiveness of Psychiatric Teaching," *American Journal of Psychiatry,* 122 (1965), 61–67.

49. Citizens Commission of Graduate Medical Education, *The Graduate Education of Physicians,* pp. 48–55.

50. Milton Mazer, "Psychiatric Disorders in General Practice: The Experience of an Island Community," *American Journal of Psychiatry,* 124 (1967), 609.

51. An active psychiatric liaison service as an integral part of psychiatric residency training can help train future psychiatrists in the process of consultation so they will be able to work most effectively with other doctors. At the same time, an active liaison service can give residents in other specialties experience in how the psychiatrist can be useful to them in their

own role as physician. An early example of active liaison work out of a department of psychiatry is described by M. Ralph Kaufman and Sydney G. Margolis, in "Theory and Practice of Psychosomatic Medicine in a General Hospital," *Medical Clinics of North America*, 32 (1948), 611–616. *See also* Harry T. Paxton, "They Have a Psychiatrist on Every Ward," *Hospital Physician* (December 1967), 46–51; Robert T. Corney, "The Efficacy of a Liaison Psychiatric Consultation Programme," *Medical Care*, 4, 3 (1966), 133–138. Avedis Donabedian stresses the still unmet need for psychiatric insights and consultations to be incorporated in patient care. He questions whether standards and strategies of care developed in teaching and research-oriented hospitals are meaningful when applied to general practice. "If parsimony is a value in medical care, the identification of redundancy becomes an element in the evaluation of care . . . when resources are limited, optimal medical care for the community may require less than 'the best' care for its individual members" ("Evaluating the Quality of Medical Care," *Milbank Memorial Fund Quarterly*, 44 [1966], 192–193).

52. Paul Barabee, "A Study of a Mental Hospital," unpub. Ph.D. diss., Harvard University, 1951, p. 222.

53. Howard S. Becker, Blanche Geer, Everett C. Hughes, and Anselm L. Strauss, *Boys in White* (Chicago: University of Chicago Press, 1961), p. 317.

54. Coser, *Life in the Ward*, p. 54.

55. Rose Coser quotes Renée Fox, *ibid.*, p. 62.

56. Marvin Scott notes: "The sociologist has been slow to take as a serious subject of investigation what is perhaps the most distinctive feature of humans—talk. . . . Future research on accounts may fruitfully take as a unit of analysis the speech community. This unit is composed of human aggregates in frequent and regular interaction. By dint of their association sharers of a distinct body of verbal signs are set off from other speech communities" (Marvin B. Scott and Stanford M. Lyman, "Accounts," *American Sociological Review*, 33 [1968], 61).

57. John J. Schwab, Roy S. Clemmons, and Leon Marder, "Training Psychiatric Residents in Consultation Work," *Journal of Medical Education*, 41 (1966), 1079.

58. Kendall, *The Relationship between Medical Educators*, pp. 41, 60.

59. In later practice, is the alumnus of a relatively lower prestige hospital "off form" when he communicates with alumni from a more prestigious hospital, as Whyte's street corner gangs were seldom "in form" when they played against high-ranking members? *See* William Foote Whyte, *Street Corner Society* (Chicago: University of Chicago Press, 1943), pp. 19–20.

60. Robert Rosenthal and Lenore Jacobson, "Self-Fulfilling Prophecies in the Classroom: Teachers' Expectations as Unintended Determinants of Pupils' Intellectual Competence," in Martin Deutsch, Irwin Katz, and Arthur R. Jensen, eds., *Social Class, Race, and Psychological Development* (New York: Holt Rinehart and Winston, 1968), pp. 219–253.

61. Lindsay E. Beaton, "A Doc Ain't Never Thru," *Journal of the*

American Medical Association, 189 (1964), 40–42; and Warren L. Bostick, "The Town-Gown Syndrome: Etiological Factors," *Journal of the American Medical Association,* 189 (1964), 113–115.

62. Kendall, *The Relationship between Medical Educators,* p. 97. *See also* the discussion of this problem that exists in universities generally in relation to their local communities in Delbert C. Miller, "Town and Gown: The Power Structure of a University Town," *American Journal of Sociology,* 68 (1963), 432–443.

63. Kendall, *The Relationship between Medical Educators,* p. 17.

64. For a discussion of the two reward systems of the "creators and purveyors" of science and their function, *see* Zetterberg, *Social Theory,* pp. 116–129; and *see* Logan Wilson, *The Academic Man* (New York: Oxford University Press, 1942), p. 16.

65. Clute, *The General Practitioner,* pp. 87, 162.

66. Webster, "Career Decisions and Professional Self-Images of Medical Students," p. 54.

67. There is evidence that the general practitioner today may not only be out of touch with recent scientific advances but also somewhat unknowing about the available services and agencies that could help their patients. The medical isolationism of some of these clinicians may extend to all aspects of their work. *See* Elaine Cumming, "The Family Doctor: Prototype of Medical Caretaker," in *Systems of Social Regulation,* with the assistance of Claire Rudolph and Laura Edell (New York: Atherton Press, 1969), pp. 30–33.

IX THE USES OF DIVERSITY

1. *See* John H. Knowles, "Medical School, Teaching Hospital, and Social Responsibility: Medicine's Clarion Call," in *The Teaching Hospital: Evolution and Contemporary Issues* (Cambridge, Mass.: Harvard University Press, 1966), pp. 100–101; and *see* Merton's discussion of inappropriate responses resulting when past training is applied to new situations in, Robert K. Merton, *Social Theory and Social Structure* (Glencoe, Ill.: The Free Press, 1957), pp. 197–200. *See also,* Max Lerner, ed., *The Portable Veblen* (New York: Viking Press, 1958), pp. 364–375, on the penalty of taking the lead.

2. *See* David Mechanic and Margaret Newton, "Social Considerations in Medical Education," *Journal of Chronic Diseases,* 18 (1965), 299; Basil R. Meyerowitz, "Current Dilemma of Medical Education in United States of America," *New York State Journal of Medicine,* 68 (1968), 449; and *see* Emile Durkheim, *Education and Sociology* (Glencoe, Ill.: The Free Press, 1956), pp. 61–90, on the social functions of education.

3. For two discussions of the variety of physicians needed for the future, *see* Edmund D. Pellegrino, "The Generalist Function in Medicine," *Journal of the American Medical Association,* 198 (1966), 541–545; and Daniel H. Funkenstein, "Implications of the Rapid Social Changes in Universities

and Medical Schools for the Education of Future Physicians," *Journal of Medical Education*, 43 (1968), 433–454. *See also* S. David Pomrinse and Bernard M. Weinstein, "Improvement of Medical Care Programs by Means of a New Type of Hospital Affiliation," *American Journal of Public Health*, 55 (1965), 1643–1652.

4. James W. Bartlett, "The Improved Preparation of Entering Medical Students: Implications for Special Placement," presented at the Annual Meeting, Group on Student Affairs, Association of American Medical Colleges, New York, October 1967. *Also see* Daniel H. Funkenstein, "The Changing Pool of Medical School Applicants," *Bulletin of the American College of Physicians*, 8 (1967), 376–382.

5. Funkenstein, "Implications of the Rapid Social Changes," p. 452.

6. Edmund D. Pellegrino, "Beehives, Mouse Traps, and Candlesticks: A Dilemma for Medical Educators," *Ohio State Medical Journal*, 59 (1963), 607.

7. Citizens Commission on Graduate Medical Education, *The Graduate Education of Physicians* (Chicago: American Medical Association, 1966), pp. 2, 4.

8. William Osler, "The Master-Word in Medicine," in *Aequanimitis with Other Addresses*, 3d ed. (Philadelphia: Blakiston Co., 1932), p. 362.

9. Articles in the lay press offer moving arguments for allowing the patient to die in peace. Yet such articles ignore the possibilities of what would follow if some physicians were not so wholeheartedly committed to saving life.

10. As we observed in Chapter VII, doing a job well sometimes requires different attributes from seeming to do the job well. The name and the action of Joseph Surface in Sheridan's *The School for Scandal* dramatize this possibility of divergence between appearance of a virtue and holding the virtue. Surface advises Lady Teazle to take a lover, urging that the lady's reputation would improve, for she would become very cautious to appear virtuous. People would have less evidence to talk about her, and she would no longer be the subject of scandal.

11. Lindsay E. Beaton, "A Doc Ain't Never Thru," *Journal of the American Medical Association*, 189 (1964), 41; and *see* Pellegrino, "Beehives, Mouse Traps," pp. 608–609.

12. Daniel H. Funkenstein, "Possible Contributions of Psychological Testing of the Nonintellectual Characteristics of Applicants to Medical School," *Journal of Medical Education*, 32, part 2 (1957), 88–112.

Robert K. Merton writes: "it is no longer a question of which type of social climate makes for more effective learning but rather a question of the extent to which the behavior of the teacher lives up to the expectations of the students, irrespective of whether these are expectations of 'authoritarian' or 'democratic' behavior" ("Notes of Problem-Finding in Sociology," in Robert K. Merton, Leonard Broom, Leonard S. Cottrell, Jr., eds., *Sociology Today* [New York: Basic Books, Inc., 1959], p. xxxii). *See also* Robert

E. Coker, Jr., Bernard G. Greenberg, and John Kosa, "Authoritarianism and Machiavellianism among Medical Students," *Journal of Medical Education,* 40 (1965), 1074–1084; Edwin B. Hutchins, "The AAMC Study of Medical Student Attrition: School Characteristics and Dropout Rate," *Journal of Medical Education,* 40 (1965), 921–927.

13. John L. Caughey, Jr., "Communications: Nonintellectual Components of Medical Education," *Journal of Medical Education,* 42 (1967), 623–624.

14. Some physicians express concern about medical research and teaching taking the central place in some hospitals and the preferment accorded research and teaching staff over clinicians. The trend thus provides most effective support for perhaps 15 percent of the doctors in training.

15. Citizens Commission on Graduate Medical Education, *The Graduate Education of Physicians,* p. 43.

16. *See* Kenneth F. Clute, *The General Practitioner: A Study of Medical Education in Ontario and Nova Scotia* (Toronto: University of Toronto Press, 1963), p. 136; and Ann Cartwright, *Patients and Their Doctors: A Study of General Practice* (New York: Atherton Press, 1967), p. 23.

17. Clute, *The General Practitioner,* p. 314.

18. Leo W. Simmons, "The Academic Lecture: A Sociologist's View of Patient Care," *American Journal of Psychiatry,* 117 (1960), 385–392.

19. Eric Hodgins, "Listen: The Patient," *New England Journal of Medicine,* 274 (1966), 658.

20. Caughey, "Communications," pp. 619–625.

21. For example, Kadushin gives abundant evidence of the need for the medical profession to take patient systems of reinforcement into consideration and work *with* it. *See* Charles Kadushin, *Why People Go to Psychiatrists* (New York: Atherton Press, 1969).

22. *See* Rue Bucher and Joan Stelling, "Characteristics of Professional Organizations," *Journal of Health and Social Behavior,* 10 (1969), 3–15.

23. Peter V. Lee, *Medical Schools and the Changing Times* (Evanston, Ill.: Association of American Medical Colleges, 1962), p. 50.

24. *See,* for example, Cecil G. Sheps, "The Medical School: Community Expectations," in Hans Popper, ed., *Trends in New Medical Schools* (New York: Grune & Stratton, 1967), p. 10; and Kurt W. Deuschle and Hugh S. Fulmer, "Community Medicine: A 'New' Department at the University of Kentucky College of Medicine," *Journal of Medical Education,* 37 (1962), 435; Robert H. Ebert, "The Role of the Medical School in Planning the Health-Care System," *Journal of Medical Education,* 42 (1967), 487. *See also* Michael J. McNamara, "A Teaching Program in Community Medicine," *Archives of Environmental Health,* 9 (1964), 807–813; Robert H. Ebert, "Medical Education and Community Needs," *Journal of Pediatrics,* 69 (1966), 876–879.

25. "The *modus operandi* of those in preventive medicine, public health, or community medicine is almost diametrically opposed to this traditional view" (Harold J. Simon, "The Medical Student: What He Wants and Needs

Versus What He Gets," *Journal of Medical Education,* 42 [1967], 777–778).

26. Arnold I. Kisch and Leo G. Reeder, "Client Evaluation of Physician Performance," *Journal of Health and Social Behavior,* 10 (1969), 56.

27. "The fact is that an informed public has already decided to devote significant part of its material resources to the purposes of better health and has expressed its will in legislation and appropriation. It promises to go much further in this direction in the future. In so doing, it regards the physician and the university as instruments of social purpose. While the initiative has not been theirs, the university and the community of practicing physicians are now impelled toward a confrontation for which they have had little time to prepare and for which there is little precedent. This confrontation will surely complicate the interrelationships of medical schools and practitioners" (Edmund D. Pellegrino, "Regionalization: An Integrated Effort of Medical School, Community, and Practicing Physician," *Bulletin of the New York Academy of Medicine,* 42 [1966], 1193). *See also* Lester J. Evans, "Preface," in Samuel W. Bloom, *The Doctor and His Patient* (New York: Russell Sage Foundation, 1963), p. 8.

28. Merlin K. DuVal, Jr., "Community and Professional Problems with a New Medical School," *Journal of The Mount Sinai Hospital,* 34 (1967), 230.

29. John Knowles notes that the "medical profession generally speaks with authority on the socio-economic problems of medicine; paradoxically, some physicians may be less widely educated on these subjects than the lay public because their education has the limitations of inbreeding and fear of change. Lest the hospital administrator enjoy this tirade, let me say that he has made no attempt to educate his staff and explain the hospital's peculiar problems" (Knowles, "Medical School," p. 90).

30. Cecil G. Sheps, Dean A. Clark, John W. Gerdes, Ethelmarie Halpern, and Nathan Hershey, "Medical Schools and Hospitals: Interdependence for Education and Service," *Journal of Medical Education,* 40, part 2 (1965), 29.

31. Kenneth E. Boulding, "The Concept of Need for Health Services," *Milbank Memorial Fund Quarterly,* 44 (October 1966), 216.

Index of Subjects

Index of Authors